Dr. John Murphy has done a splendid job of capturing the concepts and techniques of solution-focused therapy that clinicians can integrate into their therapeutic practice, regardless of their theoretical orientation. Highlighted are the collaborative relational stance, the unique strengths of this approach, and the centrality of encouraging client feedback, which are used to enhance the therapeutic process. The book is a scholarly treatise, yet the author presents the spirit of this approach in a conversational, personal, engaging, and practical way.

—**Gerald Corey, EdD, ABPP,** Distinguished Visiting Professor of Counseling, University of Holy Cross, New Orleans, LA, United States; author, *Theory and Practice of Counseling and Psychotherapy* (11th ed.)

A master at making complex concepts accessible, John Murphy provides one of the best introductions to solution focused therapy available today. His overview of the approach's history is one of the most comprehensive I've seen, and everyone will appreciate his clear explanations for putting this theory into practice. Kudos to the author for demystifying this often misunderstood theory.

—**Diane R. Gehart, PhD,** founder, Therapy that Works Institute; author, *Mastering Competencies in Family Therapy*

Solution-Focused Therapy is highly informative and well written, practical and engaging, with numerous illustrative transcripts and lots of useful supporting worksheets and guidelines. I knew Steve de Shazer and Insoo Kim Berg, the originators of SFT, and I believe that they would be very pleased with Dr. Murphy's fine contribution. Highly recommended!

—**Michael F. Hoyt, PhD,** author, *Brief Therapy and Beyond: Stories, Language, Love, Hope, and Time*; coauthor, *Brief Therapy Conversations: Exploring Efficient Intervention in Psychotherapy* (with F. Cannistrà)

John J. Murphy has always been my favorite solution-focused therapist and writer. Alongside his laser focus on client strengths, resources, and potential, he is relationally oriented. His kindness and empathy shine through in everything he writes.

—**John Sommers-Flanagan, PhD,** Professor, University of Montana, Missoula, MT, United States; coauthor, *Clinical Interviewing* (7th ed.), *Counseling and Psychotherapy Theories in Context and Practice* (3rd ed.), and several other books

Solution-Focused Therapy

Theories of Psychotherapy Series

Theories of Psychotherapy Series
Matt Englar-Carlson, Series Editor

Solution-Focused Therapy

John J. Murphy

 AMERICAN PSYCHOLOGICAL ASSOCIATION

The opinions and statements published are the responsibility of the author, and such opinions and statements do not necessarily represent the policies of the American Psychological Association.

Published by
American Psychological Association
750 First Street, NE
Washington, DC 20002
https://www.apa.org

Order Department
https://www.apa.org/pubs/books
order@apa.org

Typeset in Minion by Circle Graphics, Inc., Reisterstown, MD

Printer: Gasch Printing, Odenton, MD
Cover Designer: Beth Schlenoff Design, Bethesda, MD
Cover Art: *Lily Rising*, 2005, oil and mixed media on panel in craquelure frame, by Betsy Bauer

Library of Congress Cataloging-in-Publication Data

Names: Murphy, John J. (John Joseph), 1955- author.
Title: Solution-focused therapy / John J. Murphy.
Description: Washington, DC : American Psychological Association, [2024] |
   Series: Theories of psychotherapy series | Includes bibliographical
   references and index.
Identifiers: LCCN 2023016583 (print) | LCCN 2023016584 (ebook) |
   ISBN 9781433837678 (paperback) | ISBN 9781433837685 (ebook)
Subjects: LCSH: Solution-focused therapy. | BISAC: PSYCHOLOGY /
   Psychotherapy / Counseling | PSYCHOLOGY / Clinical Psychology
Classification: LCC RC489.S65 M87 2024 (print) | LCC RC489.S65 (ebook) |
   DDC 616.89/147--dc23/eng/20230527
LC record available at https://lccn.loc.gov/2023016583
LC ebook record available at https://lccn.loc.gov/2023016584

https://doi.org/10.1037/0000370-000

Printed in the United States of America

10 9 8 7 6 5 4 3 2 1

Contents

CONTENTS

Series Preface

Matt Englar-Carlson

Some might argue that in the contemporary clinical practice of psycho-therapy, the focus on evidence-based intervention and effective out-come has overshadowed theory in importance. Maybe. But at the same time, psychotherapists adopt and practice according to one theory or another because their experience, and decades of empirical evidence, suggests that having a sound theory of psychotherapy leads to greater therapeutic success. Theory is fundamental in guiding psychotherapists in understanding *why* people behave, think, and feel in certain ways, and it provides the guidance to then contemplate *what* a client can do to insti-gate meaningful change. Still, the role of theory in the helping process itself can be hard to explain. This narrative about solving problems may help convey theory's importance:

> Aesop tells the fable of the sun and wind having a contest to decide who was the most powerful. From above the earth, they spotted a person walking down the street, and the wind said that he bet he could get his coat off. The sun agreed to the contest. The wind blew, and the person held on tightly to his coat. The more the wind blew, the tighter the person held on to his coat. The sun said it was his turn. He put all of his energy into creating warm sunshine, and soon the person took off his coat.

What does a competition between the sun and the wind to get the person to remove a coat have to do with theories of psychotherapy? This deceptively simple story highlights the importance of theory as the precursor to any effective intervention—and hence to a favorable outcome. Without a guiding theory, a psychotherapist might treat the symptom without understanding the role of the individual. Or we might create power conflicts with our clients and not understand that, at times, indirect means of helping (sunshine) are often as effective as—if not more so than—direct ones (wind). In the absence of theory, a psychotherapist might lose track of the treatment rationale and instead get caught up in, for example, social correctness and not wanting to do something that looks too simple.

What exactly *is* theory? The *APA Dictionary of Psychology, Second Edition* defines theory as "a principle or body of interrelated principles that purports to explain or predict a number of interrelated phenomena" (VandenBos, 2015, p. 1081). In psychotherapy, a theory is a set of principles used to explain human thought and behavior, including what causes people to change. In practice, a theory frames the goals of therapy and specifies how to pursue them. Haley (1997) noted that a theory of psychotherapy ought to be simple enough for the average psychotherapist to understand but comprehensive enough to account for a wide range of eventualities. Furthermore, a theory guides action toward successful outcomes while generating hope in both the psychotherapist and client that recovery is possible.

Theory is the compass that allows psychotherapists to navigate the vast territory of clinical practice. In the same ways that navigational tools have been modified to adapt to advances in thinking and ever-expanding territories to explore, theories of psychotherapy have evolved over time to account for advances in science and technology. The different schools of theories are commonly referred to as *waves*—the first wave of psychodynamic theories (i.e., Adlerian, psychoanalytic), the second wave of learning theories (i.e., behavioral, cognitive-behavioral), the third wave of humanistic theories (i.e., person centered, gestalt, existential), the fourth wave of feminist and multicultural theories, and the fifth wave of postmodern and constructivist theories (i.e., narrative, constructivist). In many ways, these waves represent how psychotherapy has adapted and responded to changes in psychology, society, and epistemology, as well as to changes in psychotherapy itself. The wide variety of theories is also a testament to the different ways in which the same human behavior can be conceptualized depending on the view one espouses (Sommers-Flanagan & Sommers-Flanagan, 2018). Existing and emerging theories of psychotherapy are also challenged to expand beyond the primarily Western worldview endemic in most psychotherapy theories and the practice of psychotherapy itself. That revision and correction requires theories and psychotherapists to become inclusive of the full range of human diversity to reflect an understanding of human behavior that accounts for a client's context, identity, and intersectionality (American Psychological Association, 2017). To that end, psychotherapy and the theories that guide it are dynamic and responsive to the changing world around us.

With these two concepts in mind—the central importance of theory and the natural evolution of theoretical thinking—the APA Theories of Psychotherapy Series was developed. This series was created by my father (Jon Carlson) and me. Although educated in different eras, we both had a love of theory and often spent time discussing the range of complex ideas that drove each model. Even though my father identified strongly as an Adlerian and I was parented and raised from the Adlerian perspective, my father always espoused an appreciation for other theories and theorists— and that is something I picked up from him. As university faculty members teaching courses on the theories of psychotherapy, we wanted to create learning materials that highlighted the essence of the major theories for professionals and professionals in training. The titles in this series needed to include case examples showing the approach in action with clients who represented the full range of identities. Often in books on theory, the biography of the original theorist overshadows the evolution of the model. In contrast, our intent was to highlight the contemporary uses of the theories as well as their history and context—both past and present.

As this project began, we faced two immediate decisions: which theories to address and who best to present them. We assessed graduate-level theories of psychotherapy courses to see which theories are being taught, and we explored popular scholarly books, articles, and conferences to determine which theories draw the most interest. We then developed a dream list of authors from among the best minds in contemporary theoretical practice. To that end, each author in the series is one of the leading proponents of that approach as well as a knowledgeable practitioner. We asked each author to review the core constructs of the theory, bring the theory into the modern sphere of clinical practice by looking at it through a context of evidence-based practice, and clearly illustrate how the theory looks in application.

This is the 26th title in the series, and many titles are now in their second edition. Each title stands alone or can be put together with a few other titles to create materials for a course in the theories of psychotherapy. This option allows instructors to create a course featuring the approaches they believe are the most salient today. To support this end, APA Books has also developed videos for each of the approaches to demonstrate the theory in practice with a real client. Many of the videos show psychotherapy over six sessions with the same client. Contact APA Books for a complete list of available video programs (https://www.apa.org/pubs/videos).

There is a particular joy in seeing *Solution-Focused Therapy* published. I first met John Murphy in the mid-1990s when I was in graduate school. Solution-focused therapy was still emerging, and it was not an approach many of my faculty embraced because it challenged many accepted tenets of psychotherapy. In fact, I remember being told not to learn it. The approach was not new to me, however, as I remember my parents hosting the creators of solution-focused therapy, Steve de Shazer and Insoo Kim Berg, in our home many years before. Since that visit, my own interest in the approach had grown, and I wanted to learn all that I could, despite the wishes of my faculty. My father introduced me to John at a conference, and since that time John was always a trusted source for learning more about solution-focused therapy. When this series was originally proposed, solution-focused therapy was one of the original theories we suggested. At that time, psychologists were not the main proponents of the approach, and it was passed over in favor of more established, traditional models. Over the past 15 years, however, the popularity and scope of solution-focused therapy have only grown. When the opportunity came to add solution-focused therapy to the series, I knew John should be the author. My father and I both had hoped he would be the author when we originally suggested the series.

This monograph is beyond my expectations. It is well written, pragmatic, and engaging. The reader will understand the history of solution-focused therapy and why it is unique and increasingly popular. I am particularly impressed with the reader-friendly tone of the monograph. The clinical examples illustrate the approach, and the many resources allow even a novice clinician the tools needed to apply the model in practice. John Murphy has delivered a monograph clearly worth the wait.

How to Use This Book With APA Psychotherapy Videos

Each book in the Theories of Psychotherapy Series is usually paired with a video that demonstrates the theory applied in actual therapy with a real client. Many videos feature the author of the book as the guest therapist, allowing students to see an eminent scholar and practitioner putting the theory they write about into action.

The video programs have several features that make them excellent tools for learning more about theoretical concepts. Most programs have a brief introductory discussion recapping the basic features of the theory or concept being demonstrated. This allows viewers to review the key aspects of the approach about which they have just read.

Many videos feature volunteer clients in unedited psychotherapy sessions. This provides a unique opportunity to get a sense of the look and feel of real psychotherapy, something that written case examples and transcripts sometimes cannot convey. Other videos feature actors in scripted sessions that clearly illustrate the concept being presented.

The books and videos together make a powerful teaching tool for showing how theoretical principles affect practice. In the case of this book, the video *Solution-Focused Therapy in Practice* (https://www.apa.org/pubs/videos/solution-focused-therapy-practice), which features author John J. Murphy as the guest expert, provides a vivid example of how this approach looks in practice. Dr. Murphy demonstrates this approach by collaborating with a client to set a direction for therapy, build on the client's skills and resources, and construct a way forward. This powerful demonstration is framed by an informative discussion hosted by Dr. Cheri Marmarosh.

For more information, please visit APA Videos (https://www.apa.org/pubs/videos/).

Acknowledgments

I am thankful to Steve de Shazer and Insoo Kim Berg for asking, "What do clients and therapists talk about when therapy is successful?" Their answers will continue to live on in new generations of solution-focused therapists and practices. The client-directed convictions of my friend and mentor, Barry Duncan, have had a lasting impact on my work. To colleagues and students at the University of Central Arkansas, thank you for your encouragement and friendship. Current and former students, too many to name, have provided useful feedback on previous drafts of the book.

I also want to thank the American Psychological Association, series editor Matt Englar-Carlson, and development editor Molly Gage for their feedback on an earlier version of the manuscript and their enthusiasm about the transcultural promise and possibilities of solution-focused therapy. It is a privilege to contribute to a book series that includes works by many authors I have studied and admired over the years. Words fall short in expressing my appreciation for my family—Deb, Tom, Helen, Erin, Corey, Maura, Robbie, Ruby, Julia, Dottie, and Millie (the list keeps growing). To workshop participants throughout the world, thank you for your kindness, questions, and commitment to client-centered care. As always, I am indebted to my clients for their ongoing patience and lessons on how to be useful.

Solution-Focused
Therapy

1

Introduction

Trey entered the office cautiously and took a seat across the table from me.[1] He glanced around the room at the bookshelves, wall hangings, and a few other items—anything but me. Trey, a 9-year-old African American student in an inner-city elementary school, was referred by his teachers for a psychoeducational evaluation due to academic problems. As the school psychologist, I was required to complete a social history interview and form at the start of every evaluation, which typically took about 5 minutes. As it turns out, my conversation with Trey that day was anything but typical.

After a few introductory comments, I asked who he lived with at home. "My aunt and five cousins," Trey replied. His school file stated that he had been removed from his mother's custody the previous year due to child abuse and that his father died when Trey was 6. When I told him I was sorry about his father's passing, he quietly told me his father

---

[1] In all clinical case material in this book identities have been disguised and other steps have been taken to protect client confidentiality.

https://doi.org/10.1037/0000370-001
Solution-Focused Therapy, by J. J. Murphy

was murdered by "a guy named George" in the kitchen of their apartment. "They were yelling, and George shot him. The police came and took George away, and they took me to my aunt's house." The social history interview had taken an unexpected turn.

"I bet it's hard not seeing your dad," I said. Trey nodded and described other struggles involving various family members. He had two older brothers named James and Robert. James was in prison and Robert was on probation. Trey had been in three different schools during the past 3 years. After telling me his aunt might move again, he put his face in his hands and sobbed.

We sat in silence for a minute or so before I noticed a few tears collecting on the table under Trey's face. I was at a loss for words. We sat for another minute, Trey with his face in his hands and me staring a hole in the table. I couldn't shake the idea that Trey had suffered more in 9 years than some people do in a lifetime.

I finally broke the silence. "With everything you've been through, how do you keep hanging in there and coming to school?"

Trey looked at me for the first time and said, "My aunt always tells me to never give up because quitters don't make it."

I followed his lead by asking, "What else does she say or do that helps you?"

Trey replied, "She's always saying, 'try hard,' 'do your best,' and stuff like that. And that I'd be the first one in the family to graduate from high school."

When asked what else kept him going, Trey described several coping skills and other resources. I felt myself becoming more hopeful, and Trey seemed more energized as the conversation shifted from what was wrong or lacking in his life to what was right and working. He spoke faster and with more expression. He leaned forward, held his head higher, and made more eye contact. Among other things, I learned that his brother Robert occasionally helped him with homework and that he did better in math when teachers gave him more time to complete class work. I thanked him for talking with me and walked him back to class.

Trey and I completed the evaluation a few weeks later, and my report included the following recommendations taken directly from our previous conversation: additional homework help from Robert, extra time for math work in class, tutoring from older students at school, and continued encouragement from his aunt. Although I did not think of it in these terms at the time, every suggestion was built on what was already available and working in Trey's life—his ideas, social supports, and other indigenous strengths and resources in his life.

I began to search for a more systematic way to initiate collaborative, client-directed, strengths-based conversations like the first one with Trey. The search led to a small group of clinicians in Milwaukee, led by Steve de Shazer and Insoo Kim Berg, who were experimenting with an innovative brief therapy approach. They called it "solution-focused" brief therapy to highlight the emphasis on what clients wanted from therapy and what they were already doing or already had in their lives that would help toward achieving it. This book uses the shorter term *solution-focused therapy* (SFT) to capture the approach's essence and distinguish it from problem-focused approaches that have dominated the psychotherapy profession for over a century.

WHAT IS SOLUTION-FOCUSED THERAPY?

SFT is a collaborative approach that invites clients[2] to describe what they want from therapy and apply what they already have in place toward achieving it in the shortest time possible. Therapists are guided by three self-talk questions:

- What does the client want from therapy?
- What does the client already have toward achieving it?
- What progress has the client already made and what are some possible next signs or next steps toward further progress?

---

[2]In this book, the term *clients* refers to individuals, couples, families, or other therapy participants. *Therapists* and *practitioners* include psychotherapists, psychiatrists, counselors, social workers, and other service providers. *Therapist* is used in client illustrations and dialogues for the sake of consistency. *Solutions* refers to positive steps toward desired outcomes rather than ideal outcomes or absence of problems.

These questions translate into the following three main tasks of SFT:

1. *Setting a direction* on the basis of what the client wants from therapy: What are your best hopes from talking with me? How would your life be different if you achieved those hopes?
2. *Building on exceptions and other resources* that are already happening and available in the client's life: When is/was the problem less noticeable? Tell me about a time your best hopes have happened. How did you make that happen? What/who else might help you move closer to your best hopes?
3. *Exploring progress* toward desired outcomes: What's better since we last met? How did you move up on the 0–10 scale? What might be the next small sign/step toward further progress?

These tasks represent the entirety of SFT and occur in varying degrees and sequences during most sessions.

The *three main techniques* of SFT are *asking, listening,* and *amplifying.* Therapists ask useful questions, listen closely to clients' responses, and amplify aspects of their responses and lives that support desired outcomes. When being purely solution-focused, there is rarely anything else the therapist does outside of these activities. The definition of SFT highlights several key features. SFT is:

Collaborative

SFT is a collaborative, client-directed approach that invites clients to participate in every aspect of therapy to the extent they are willing and able to do so. In contrast to approaches in which therapists prescribe interventions based on their expertise and theoretical perspective, solution-focused therapists elicit solutions from clients by approaching them from a position of humility and "not knowing" (H. Anderson, 2007).

Assuming a stance of not knowing does not mean relinquishing one's expertise or influence. As Weakland (1993) noted, "Influence is inherent in all human interaction. . . . The only choice is between doing so without reflection, or even with attempted denial, and doing so deliberately and responsibly" (p. 143). Microanalysis research indicates that therapists of all orientations influence the content of conversation by deciding what to ask and not ask, what to follow up on and let go, and so forth (Bavelas et al., 2014). In SFT, these decisions are guided by the client's goals and responses rather than the therapist's preferences. As Iveson et al. (2012) said, the therapist "would rather be invisible than significant; someone who generates and manages a conversation in which the client hears his or her own words either for the first time or with fresh ears" (p. 127).

Invitational

When SFT practitioners ask questions or offer suggestions, they are presented as *invitations* rather than directives. For a client who reported recent improvements, the therapist might offer the following suggestion: "It may be helpful to watch for small signs of progress. How does that sound to you?" The invitational tone is conveyed by the phrase, "It *may* be helpful" and the question, "How does that sound *to you*?" Presenting questions and suggestions in this manner encourages clients to freely accept, reject, or modify them as needed with no pressure or pushback from the therapist.

Descriptive

Solution-focused therapists elicit descriptions of client hopes, resources, and progress rather than interpreting client actions, motives, and feelings. Consider the following detail-gathering sequence of questions: "What will you notice first when things get a little better? Then what? Who else will notice? How might they respond? What will that be like for you?" Although this sequence of questions lacks the most important element of the conversation—the client's response—it briefly illustrates SFT's emphasis on description.

Focused on What Clients Want

Focusing on what clients want *more* of (vs. less of) is why SFT is considered an *addition* (vs. subtraction) approach. The entire SFT process revolves around what the client wants from therapy, which is addressed at the very outset of services ("What are your best hopes from this? What will be different to tell you it was useful?"). Asking what clients want from therapy neither denies the problem nor prohibits clients from discussing problems—it simply invites them to focus on what they want *instead*. This phase of SFT is referred to as *formulating goals* or *setting a direction*.[3] Regardless of one's terminology, the first and most important task of SFT is to determine what the client wants from it.

Focused on What Clients Have

Instead of assuming that client problems indicate personal deficiencies, solution-focused therapists assume clients possess the resources needed to improve their lives. This does not imply that clients would not benefit from additional knowledge and skills. It just means that SFT focuses on helping them build solutions from what is already available and working in their lives—strengths, attributes, successes, social supports, and other resources that can help them achieve hoped-for outcomes.

Brief (Shortest Time Possible)

SFT is brief by design versus default, and every session is approached as if it were the last. This practical mindset expedites change by keeping therapists and clients on track. It also explains why SFT techniques are commonly used in single-session therapy (Hoyt et al., 2018). The "brief" component of SFT does not mean clients are rushed into action or therapists are insensitive to their struggles. Brevity is more of a by-product than a goal of SFT. Therapists rarely set a preestablished limit on the length of therapy

---

[3] I prefer the terms *desired* (or *hoped-for*) *outcome*, *preferred future*, and *setting a direction* to the more conventional language of "goals and goal setting" because they effectively portray the SFT process of helping clients describe what they want from therapy and scale their movement and progress toward achieving it. If you prefer goal-based language or are required to use it for documentation purposes, then you can view the client's desired outcome as a general goal, the preferred future as a detailed goal, and setting a direction as goal setting.

because that decision, like others, is made in close collaboration with clients. Agencies and therapists that have used SFT for many years have estimated the average length of therapy to be 3 to 6.5 sessions (Macdonald, 2017). Perhaps the most practical guideline for determining the length of therapy was offered by de Shazer, who said "as long as it takes and not one session more" (as cited in Ratner et al., 2012).

Although most therapists do not think of themselves as brief therapists, research suggests they are doing "unplanned brief therapy" (10 sessions or fewer) regardless of their preferences, theoretical orientation, or training (Levenson, 2017). It appears that clients will either achieve their therapeutic goals during that time or drop out if they don't (Muran et al., 2009; Wierzbicki & Pekarik, 1993). These findings suggest that therapists do not have much of a choice as to whether or not to do brief therapy. The choice is whether to do so by design or default. The fact that SFT has always been brief by design—in combination with its evidence base and multicultural orientation—helps to explain its increased popularity among therapists and clients throughout the world (Neipp & Beyebach, 2022). Since most clients prefer as few sessions as possible, it seems respectful to honor that preference regardless of one's therapy approach.

SFT AND EVIDENCE-BASED PRACTICE

In 2005, the American Psychological Association (APA) established the Task Force on Evidence-Based Practice to define evidence-based practice in psychotherapy and other psychological services. The task force was made up of scientists and practitioners from diverse theoretical perspectives. Their work resulted in a tripartite definition of evidence-based practice as "the integration of the best available research with clinical expertise in the context of patient characteristics, culture, and preferences" (APA Task Force on Evidence-Based Practice, 2006, p. 273). Since this is part of an APA book series, it seems fitting to address the compatibility between SFT and the three main features of evidence-based practice—research-informed practice; clinical expertise; and client characteristics, culture, and preferences.

Research-Informed Practice

Research and evidence-based practice have played a key role in SFT throughout its history. From the late 1970s to the present, the approach has been examined in descriptive studies, randomized controlled trials, microanalyses, and meta-analytic reviews of outcome studies. These investigations provide extensive evidence of SFT's widespread effectiveness across a variety of clients, countries, and problems (Neipp & Beyebach, 2022).

SFT is also responsive to the well-researched "common factors" of effective psychotherapy. Decades of research have confirmed that the success of any therapy approach depends largely on the extent to which it activates common factors such as client involvement, resources, hope, and feedback—all of which are central in solution-focused practice (Kort et al., 2021).

SFT has also been listed on several federal and state registries of evidence-based practice in the United States. For example, it has been recognized as a promising approach by the Substance Abuse and Mental Health Services Administration's National Registry of Evidence-Based Programs and Practices and the Office of Juvenile Justice and Delinquency Prevention (Kim et al., 2019). Unfortunately, these federal registries were closed due to lack of funding before they could review more compelling evidence of SFT's effectiveness from the past decade. The approach has also been listed as an evidence-based practice by the Oregon Health Authority Addiction and Mental Health Services department (2017). Solution-based casework, which includes many features of SFT, was designated a "promising intervention" by the California Evidence-Based Clearinghouse for Child Welfare (2022). Beyond these formal recognitions, SFT has been widely taught and formally recognized as an effective approach by accreditation programs, universities, and training institutes in many countries throughout the world.

As with any therapy approach, there is a continued need for well-designed studies of SFT with a diverse range of cultures, concerns, and clients, including clients of underrepresented racial/ethnic backgrounds and intersectional identities. Cross-cultural research reviews and meta-analyses have verified SFT's credibility as a transcultural, evidence-based psychotherapy that works as well as other approaches in fewer sessions (Beyebach et al., 2021; Neipp & Beyebach, 2022). The efficiency and transcultural evidence base of SFT have increased its usefulness and appeal in community mental health centers, hospitals, outpatient clinics, schools, and private practice settings throughout the world. Chapter 5 examines the empirical evaluation of SFT in more detail.

Clinical Expertise

Clinical expertise in SFT requires the therapist to *ask* useful questions, *listen* to the answers, and construct follow-up questions that invite clients to *amplify* their responses by providing more details. There is rarely anything a solution-focused therapist does outside of these activities.

Although questions are a part of every therapy approach, they are particularly important in SFT. Rather than telling clients what to do, therapists ask questions that encourage clients to tell themselves. The main purpose of questions in most therapeutic approaches is to provide the clinician with information needed to devise diagnoses, interpretations, and interventions. In contrast, solution-focused questions invite clients to describe their "preferred futures" (Ratner et al., 2012) in *their* own words and *their* own way.

The approach's client-directed nature is exemplified by the fact that most of the questions therapists ask are constructed from the client's previous answers and often incorporate the client's exact words. As important as questions are in SFT, their usefulness depends entirely on the client's response. Solution-focused therapists listen with a constructive ear (Lipchik, 2002) tuned to hints of hope, strength, success, and other aspects of clients and their lives that support desired outcomes.

Client Characteristics, Culture, and Preferences

The third component of evidence-based practice emphasizes the importance of tailoring therapy to the unique characteristics, culture, and preferences of each client. Solution-focused therapists address this by customizing services to the client rather than requiring them to buy into the therapist's preferred interventions and interpretations. This involves adopting a position of cultural humility; requesting and accommodating client perceptions, preferences, and feedback; and building practical solutions from clients' indigenous strengths and resources. These features of SFT enhance the therapist's ability to provide socially just, culturally responsive services to all clients, including underrepresented persons of various racial/ethnic backgrounds and intersectional identities.

The main tasks and techniques of SFT reflect core recommendations and best practices in multiculturalism and diversity-competent practice (De Jong & Berg, 2013). Starting therapy by asking clients what they want from it—instead of diagnosing them and telling them what they need—sets a collaborative tone for everything that follows. Continuing to anchor questions and conversations to client hopes, resources, and progress further guards against cultural imperialism and other disrespectful practices. The cultural responsiveness of SFT is also reflected by the fact that it continues to grow and flourish in an increasingly wide range of cultures, countries, and client populations around the world (Beyebach et al., 2021; Kim et al., 2019; Neipp & Beyebach, 2022).

THE REST OF THE STORY

Although Trey did not qualify for special education services, he needed additional assistance at school. Building on the exceptions and other resources from our first meeting, I worked with Trey, his teachers, and his aunt to amplify what was already helping him to persevere in school and elsewhere. His math teacher agreed to provide extra time for him to complete class work when possible. Robert stepped up his efforts to help Trey with homework. His aunt was pleasantly surprised to hear about the impact of her homespun sayings and agreed to continue offering words of encouragement. Trey and I also cobbled a few of his aunt's sayings into self-talk strategies he could use as needed.

Trey continued to struggle academically, though not as much as he had before. At the end of the school year, he proudly informed me that he was promoted to the fourth grade. I congratulated him on his hard work and success. Trey taught me a valuable lesson that continues to inform and inspire my work as a solution-focused therapist: *Every client offers a one-of-a-kind set of life experiences and resources that can be applied toward therapeutic solutions.*

History

Historically psychotherapy has concerned itself with problems
(variously defined) and solutions (seldom defined at all), with the
problems receiving the major share of the effort.

—Steve de Shazer, 1988, p. 6

It was the mid-1970s in Milwaukee, Wisconsin. The beer business was booming in the blue-collar city that hosted the largest collection of breweries in the United States. But beer wasn't the only thing brewing. A small group of clinicians and researchers, led by Steve de Shazer and Insoo Kim Berg, were dissatisfied with the status quo of psychotherapy. They started meeting in de Shazer's apartment to view and discuss videotapes of their therapy sessions and eventually opened the Brief Family Therapy Center (BFTC) in downtown Milwaukee. The BFTC worked primarily with underrepresented individuals and families struggling with poverty, substance misuse, and other major challenges.

https://doi.org/10.1037/0000370-002
Solution-Focused Therapy, by J. J. Murphy

The center quickly developed a reputation for working with so-called resistant clients and multiproblem situations, often achieving successful results in a short time. The Milwaukee group spent countless hours over the next 10 years analyzing therapy sessions and developing the foundational ideas and methods of the solution-focused approach. Before discussing the group's discoveries and breakthroughs, it is useful to consider the key origins and influences of solution-focused therapy (SFT).

ORIGINS AND EARLY INFLUENCES

People have been talking with each other about their hopes and problems for centuries. This makes it practically impossible to describe the full lineage of SFT or any therapy approach developed during the late 20th century—100 years or more after Mesmer, Breuer, Freud, and others began offering the "talking cure" to people experiencing psychological problems. With these points in mind, several key individuals, ideas, and practices have strongly influenced SFT, as described next.

Milton H. Erickson

Each person is a unique individual. Hence, psychotherapy should be formulated to meet the uniqueness of the individual's needs, rather than tailoring the person to fit the Procrustean bed of a hypothetical theory.
(Milton H. Erickson, as cited in Zeig, 1982, p. vi)

The developers of SFT were strongly influenced by the ideas and methods of Milton H. Erickson (1901–1980). Erickson is considered one of the most innovative and effective practitioners in the history of psychotherapy. Although he died in 1980, his therapy methods live on through ongoing discussions of his work in books and training workshops throughout the world. Among Erickson's many contributions to the psychotherapy profession, the following are particularly relevant to SFT.

Strengths/Resources Orientation

A psychiatrist by training, Erickson believed every client offered a unique set of strengths, life experiences, and other resources that could be leveraged to help them resolve problems and enrich their lives. His unwavering faith in people's capabilities and resilience was influenced by the challenges he faced as a child and beyond (Haley, 1967). Childhood difficulties included color-blindness, tone-deafness, and dyslexia. At age 17, he was almost entirely paralyzed by polio. One day, he overheard a team of doctors tell his mother he would not overcome the paralysis and might not live through the night. Outraged that they would say such a thing, young Milton was determined to live through the night. He awoke the next morning and embarked on a demanding exercise routine that eventually enabled him to stand, balance, and put one foot in front of the other. Erickson's physical challenges persisted throughout his life, as did his confidence and efforts to overcome them and move forward.

Drawing from his own struggles and resiliency, Erickson had an abiding trust in clients' ability to move forward in the face of obstacles and difficulties (Lankton & Lankton, 1983). He viewed clients as stuck versus sick and avoided adopting any specific theories of personality or psychopathology. He believed clients did the best they could under the circumstances and acted in ways that made sense to them at a particular time or moment. Rather than conducting diagnostic assessments of clients' deficiencies, he identified what was important and available to them and encouraged them to use what they already had in their lives to move forward and achieve their goals.

Erickson's *utilization of client resources* is perhaps the most renowned feature of his work (Short et al., 2005). Instead of trying to give clients something they did not have, he invited them to apply existing values, skills, and other resources toward creative solutions. For example, he encouraged a man who claimed to be Jesus Christ to work in a local carpentry shop as a way of reestablishing social connections with others. In treating a couple who enjoyed maintaining their garden, he used gardening terms in therapy sessions and explored how their gardening expertise might help them improve their relationship. These and more examples can be found in *Uncommon Therapy*, Haley's classic book on Erickson's approach to psychotherapy (1973). Encouraging clients to apply their strengths and resources toward solutions is a core component of SFT.

Emphasis on Small Changes

Erickson encouraged clients to make small changes based on the systemic notion that one small change may lead to another, then another, and so on. He viewed therapy as a process of "tipping the first domino." In describing Erickson's work, Haley (1973) said he

> seeks a small change and enlarges upon it. If the change is in a crucial area, what appears small can change the whole system. Sometimes he uses the analogy of a hole in a dam; it does not take a very large hole to lead to a change in the structure of the whole dam. (p. 35)

SFT reflects Erickson's focus on small changes by inviting clients to notice and describe small exceptions to the problem and small signs of further progress.

Focus on Future Solutions

A trained hypnotherapist, Erickson developed a hypnotic intervention called the *crystal ball technique*. He would invite clients to envision a problem-free future as if they were watching it in a crystal ball and to describe how they resolved the problems that were blocking them from that future. Since the solutions clients described were of their own making instead of someone else's, they were more likely to implement them in their everyday lives. Sometimes this was all that was needed for a client to make useful changes. The crystal ball technique was a precursor to SFT's miracle question: "Suppose that one night, while you were asleep, there was a miracle and this problem was solved. How would you know? What would be different?" (de Shazer, 1988, p. 5).[1]

---

[1] It is impossible to pinpoint the exact origin or originator of a therapy idea or technique. The miracle question is a case in point. Although Erickson is the most immediate source given de Shazer's familiarity with his work, renowned psychotherapist Alfred Adler (1870–1937) used two similar techniques decades earlier. The first, referred to as "the question," asked clients how their lives would be different if the problem was gone. The second technique invited clients to act "as if" they did not have the problem as a way of encouraging them to adopt new ways of thinking and behaving. Adler got the idea from Hans Vaihinger's 1924 book, *The Philosophy of "As If."* It is unclear who or what may have inspired Vaihinger.

No General Client, No General Theory

Although Erickson was trained in psychoanalysis like most psychiatrists of his era, he found it to be of little practical value in helping people change. As his work became better known, therapists would often inquire about his general theory of psychopathology or psychotherapy. Erickson answered that he did not have a general theory because he had never met a general client. Following Erickson's lead, solution-focused therapists do not embrace any psychological theories about clients' personalities or problems.

Efficiency

Erickson demonstrated that meaningful and lasting therapeutic change can occur in the absence of information about the origins and history of the client's problem—which is why he is considered a pioneer of brief therapy approaches. Although his clients often made significant improvements in a short time, brevity was more of a by-product than a goal of his approach—just as it is in SFT.

Lankton and Lankton (1983) listed the following assumptions and guidelines underlying Erickson's work, all of which are evident in SFT: People make the best choice for themselves at any given moment; respect all messages from the client; never attempt to take away client choice; the resources that clients need lie within their own personal history; meet the client at their model of the world; explanations, theories, or metaphors used to describe a person are not the person; if it's hard work, break it down to smaller steps.

The impact of Erickson's work on early versions of SFT is evident in a comment by de Shazer (1982): "It was through BFTC's efforts to apply Erickson's methods and procedures that our approach was developed" (p. 28). To learn more about Erickson and his work, the Milton H. Erickson Foundation in Phoenix, Arizona, offers an abundance of books, videos, training materials, and additional resources that are listed online (https://www.erickson-foundation.org). Erickson's unique approach to psychotherapy is thoroughly described and illustrated in *Uncommon Therapy* (Haley, 1973) and *Hope and Resiliency,* a book coauthored by two of Erickson's daughters (Short et al., 2005).

Systems Theory

Prior to the 1950s, most forms of psychotherapy focused on the inner world of clients. The emergence of systems theory in the mid-20th century offered an alternative to the prevailing medical/disease model in which client problems were seen as symptoms of internal pathology. Systems theory offered the contrasting idea that individuals and problems are embedded in and inseparable from their social contexts. The systemic perspective had a particularly strong impact on family therapy and postmodern approaches such as collaborative language systems therapy (H. Anderson, 2007), narrative therapy (Madigan, 2019), and SFT (de Shazer et al., 2021).

Systemic Principles and Origins

The systemic or interactional perspective (hereinafter *systemic perspective*) evolved from two main sources: general systems theory (von Bertalanffy, 1968) and cybernetics (Weiner, 1948). Both theories challenged the scientific reductionism of the early 20th century by proposing that human processes and functioning—and humans themselves—are best understood by analyzing mutually influential relationships and inter-actions. Bronfenbrenner's (1979) ecological systems theory reinforced the powerful role (for better or worse) of social contexts and networks—particularly connections between a family or individual and the broader contexts in which they live, such as neighborhoods, countries, social and political environments, and other contexts.

Communication Research

The systemic perspective was a driving force in the communication research of Jackson, Bateson, Weakland, Watzlawick, Bavelas, and others at the Mental Research Institute (MRI) in Palo Alto, California. This research initially focused on patterns of communication between family members and was eventually expanded to therapist–client interactions. These studies led to several influential ideas and outcomes, two of which were particularly relevant to the development of SFT.

After studying the language and interactional patterns in families of persons with schizophrenia, MRI published their findings in a classic paper entitled, "Toward a Theory of Schizophrenia" (Bateson et al., 1956). One prominent finding was the powerful link between a person's behavior and their interactions and conversations with key people in their lives. Although some therapists reduced this finding to merely another type of client or family pathology, others pursued the possibility that therapist–client conversations could be deliberately designed to enhance clients' well-being and therapy outcomes. Among the latter group were social constructionists Sheila McNamee and Kenneth Gergen (McNamee & Gergen, 1992)—and SFT cofounders de Shazer and Berg.

Janet Bavelas, MRI researcher and coauthor of the classic book *Pragmatics of Human Communication* (Watzlawick et al., 1967), extended the study of communication in therapy by conducting microanalyses of client–therapist conversations in SFT and other therapy approaches. Bavelas et al. (2000) discovered two fundamentally different patterns of communication. First, there are approaches that shape therapeutic processes and conversations toward identifying pathology and toward the therapist's theories about problems and solutions (Category 1). Second, there are approaches that steer therapeutic processes and conversations toward client strengths, opinions, and other resources connected to the client's goal (Category 2). The researchers also found that all therapists used questions and formulations to preserve, delete, or transform the client's original statements. Therapists in Category 1 asked questions and formulated clients' statements in ways that accentuated clients' pathology and confirmed the therapist's theoretical orientation. Therapists in Category 2 used questions and formulations that accentuated clients' preexisting strengths and resources and preserved a large amount of their original statements. Solution-focused therapists consistently fell into Category 2.

The communication research at MRI influenced the Milwaukee group's subsequent research and development of SFT, as did the MRI brief therapy model described next.

MRI Brief Therapy Model

We find that in deliberate intervention into human problems the most pragmatic approach is not to question why? but what?; that is, what is being done here and now that serves to perpetuate the problem, and what can be done here and now to effect a change. (Watzlawick et al., 1974, p. 86)

SFT cofounders Berg and de Shazer met in the mid-1970s while visiting MRI's Brief Therapy Center to learn more about their evolving brief therapy model. The beginnings and foundations of the model were described in the book *Change: Principles of Problem Formation and Problem Resolution* (Watzlawick et al., 1974). The book included a foreword by Milton Erickson and incorporated ideas from philosophy, mathematics, systems theory, and communication theory.

The Brief Therapy Center was established in 1966 by a team of clinicians and researchers led by Paul Watzlawick, John Weakland, and Richard Fisch. Early versions of their model were strongly influenced by systems theory, communication theory, and observations of Erickson's work. As time went on, their techniques began to emerge from observations, recordings, and analyses of their own therapy sessions. Although recording and analyzing therapy sessions is commonplace today, it was uncommon and innovative at the time.

After almost a decade of work, the team proposed two core principles that guided their approach. First, they proposed that most client concerns began as ordinary life difficulties and became "problems" after the client or others persistently applied the same ineffective solution attempts (the principle of problem formation). Second, successful therapy interrupted repetitive problem patterns and encouraged clients to do something different instead of "more of the same" (the principle of problem resolution). The second MRI book, *The Tactics of Change* (Fisch et al., 1982), took up where *Change* left off by describing the nuts and bolts of MRI brief therapy through practical illustrations involving a variety clients and concerns.

The brief therapy model differed sharply from psychodynamic therapies that involved lengthy assessments and prolonged treatments. MRI clinicians began therapy by obtaining a concrete description of the problem

("Who is doing what to whom, and how is it a problem?") and then encouraged anyone involved to change one or more aspects of their typical response to the problem (Fisch et al., 1982). For example, if a couple complained of frequent arguments, they might be encouraged to whisper their next argument or write out their main points in a letter to one another. Small changes often led to larger changes and eventual problem resolution, which usually occurred in 10 sessions or fewer.

Textbook descriptions of the model frequently highlight its more dramatic and strategic elements, such as encouraging clients to do the unexpected or opposite of what they've been doing in response to the problem. Unfortunately, these descriptions overlook the approach's most important contribution as captured by Weakland's response to the question "What is the most important thing a therapist has to learn?":

> It's going to sound dreadfully simple, but it is also very difficult to do; and that is really listen to what the client says and how they say it; really listen which means a number of things. One of the main things it means is, don't get into the business of being so perceptive that you know what the client says or means better than the client does . . . it is very hard to do. . . . I am afraid that a lot of training is about being perceptive and I think it is very dangerous. It is much more important to listen. (as cited in Cade, 2007, p. 40)

MRI therapists resisted the urge to be "perceptive" in the sense of going beyond what the client said by making interpretations or assumptions based on one's previous clients, professional experiences, or theoretical model. They accepted what the client said at face value and addressed their stated concerns (Cade, 2007). They believed therapists were ethically obligated to help people resolve problems as quickly as possible, and that anything beyond that was unnecessary and unhelpful. The team summarized their approach in three practical guidelines for therapists and clients:

- Guideline 1. If it's not broken, don't fix it.
- Guideline 2. If it doesn't work, do something different.
- Guideline 3. If it works, do more of it.

These guidelines inspired SFT's emphasis on efficiency, pragmatism, and client resources. Guideline 1 urged therapists to focus on the client's stated complaint and goal and nothing beyond that. Guideline 2 addressed the common tendency of clients *and* therapists to repeat "more of the same" solution attempts despite their ineffectiveness. As described shortly, Guideline 3 became a central theme of SFT. Refer to Fisch et al. (2010) for selected MRI papers and Schlanger et al. (2019) for an updated description and application of MRI's brief therapy model.

Solution-Focused Brief Therapy: The Milwaukee Group

Where you stand determines what you see and what you do not see; . . . a change in where you stand changes everything. (Steve de Shazer, 1991, pp. xx–xxi)

In the mid-1970s, de Shazer invited his colleague (and future wife) Insoo Kim Berg to join him in his hometown of Milwaukee to build on what they had learned at MRI. Within a few months, they were meeting regularly with a small group of colleagues from diverse clinical backgrounds such as family therapy, behavioral psychology, and psychodynamic therapy. Most meetings involved analyzing each other's videotaped therapy sessions with attention to the question "What do therapists and clients talk about when therapy is successful?" In 1978, they pooled their resources and opened the BFTC in downtown Milwaukee. They quickly developed a reputation for working successfully with underrepresented clients and families struggling with poverty, substance misuse, and other significant challenges.

Berg's comments in an interview about BFTC's early years (Smith, 2006) capture the team's excitement about observations and discoveries that would become core foundations of solution-focused theory and practice: "I think in about 1980 or 1981, we started noticing that we were doing something very differently, but we didn't know what it was" (p. 3). They started a newsletter and began to host visitors who wanted to observe their work. As Berg (Smith, 2006) further recalled,

> the visitors would keep saying . . . our way of working was a bit different from the MRI method. . . . The first thing that we recognized

was different and that became part of solution focused therapy was the concept of exceptions, and that was the beginning of the whole evolution of solution focused therapy. We first noticed that we were commenting on solutions instead of problems in 1982, and then after that things started just growing, bursting out. (pp. 3–4)

Although the Milwaukee group initially focused on effective therapist behaviors and interventions, they gradually broadened their focus to client–therapist interactions associated with effective outcomes (de Shazer, 1991). They never wavered from rigorously evaluating and revising their approach in response to new observational data and discoveries. They kept what worked and discarded what didn't, a practice that highlighted SFT's emphasis on pragmatism, simplicity, and minimalism.

Many solution-focused techniques began as a spontaneous question or suggestion developed on the spot for a specific client. If a technique worked well with other clients and problems, then the group would continue to implement and evaluate it. As Trepper and Franklin (2012) noted, solution-focused practice has developed in an evidence-based manner from the very start. The BFTC's inductive, evidence-based process of research and practice resulted in a collaborative clinical style and the following realizations.

Nothing Happens All the Time

The Milwaukee group's realization that nothing happens all the time, while hardly profound, had profound implications for SFT. Regardless of the problem being discussed, clients occasionally mentioned times when it was absent or less bothersome than usual. Rather than passing these times off as flukes or random events as clients often did if they noticed them at all, the group saw them as solutions that were already happening, just not as often as preferred. They called them exceptions to the problem or *exceptions* for short (de Shazer, 1985).

Therapists invited clients to notice small exceptions as they went about their everyday lives. They explored exception-related details ("What? When? Where?") with special attention to the client's contribution ("How did you make it happen?"), personal and social consequences ("How did your partner react? What was that like for you?"), and other details and differences that distinguished exceptions from other times ("What else was different about that time?"). The focus of therapy shifted from reducing problems to increasing solutions by encouraging clients to do more of what was already working. Building on exceptions became the straightest and most efficient path to successful outcomes. Therapy became briefer and clients became more hopeful when they realized they were already being successful. Building on exceptions became a core SFT technique that exemplified the approach's emphasis on simplicity and efficiency. It also challenged long-standing problem-focused precepts and practices in psychotherapy.

Clients Know Best

The Milwaukee group came to view clients as experts on themselves and their lives. They trusted that clients knew what they wanted from therapy and had the resources needed to improve their lives. They accepted clients' goals and perceptions at face value and rarely offered advice or interpretations—choosing instead to listen carefully and ask questions about what clients wanted from therapy and what was already available and working in their lives to help them achieve it (de Shazer, 1991). Rather than focusing on the client's problem, they focused on what the client wanted instead (solution description).

They collaborated with clients on everything from formulating therapy goals to deciding when to end services (de Shazer, 1991). Centralizing clients in these ways improved outcomes and promoted collaborative therapeutic relationships. It also enhanced clients' ownership of improvements and eliminated so-called client resistance—a term the group deemed disrespectful to clients and detrimental to therapeutic outcomes (de Shazer, 1984).

Language (and Dialogue) Is Powerful

The group also discovered that successful outcomes were linked to specific client–therapist language and conversations. This discovery fueled their interest in the therapeutic possibilities of dialogue and led to the realization that a different kind of language was needed to shift from resolving problems to building solutions (de Shazer, 1994). They coined the term "solution talk" to distinguish it from the problem talk of other therapies. Solution talk centered on clients' hopes and strengths instead of their deficits and limitations. The group emphasized that solution talk was *not* about being positive, upbeat, or anything else clients might perceive as invalidating the seriousness or pain of the problem.

Drawing from their own observations and from postmodern social constructionism theory (McNamee & Gergen, 1992), the team increasingly acknowledged the role of language, dialogue, and coconstruction of meaning in SFT. Berg and de Shazer (1993) observed that as the "client and therapist talk more and more about the solution they want to construct together, they come to believe in the truth or reality of what they are talking about" (p. 9). The better clients were at describing their goals in vivid detail, the more likely they were to achieve them. They came to view the therapy conversation as the most by powerful intervention of all, and trusted clients to apply the conversation in ways that were most useful and fitting for them.

The postmodern ideas and methods described above were a radical departure from the modernist, problem-focused tenets and techniques that had dominated the field of psychotherapy for nearly a century. It is not surprising that many therapists were skeptical when they first heard or read about the approach, which is why it has taken SFT longer than other approaches to achieve credibility as a legitimate psychotherapy despite ample evidence of its effectiveness. Refer to Cade (2007) and Lipchik et al. (2012) for additional information on the early history of SFT and the Milwaukee group's work at the BFTC.

Other Contributors

The steady growth of SFT has resulted not only from the writings of de Shazer and Berg but also from the contributions of many others within and outside the original Milwaukee group—a few of whom are noted next.

Lipchik

A family therapist and core member of the original Milwaukee group, Eve Lipchik left the BFTC in 1988 to start a private practice. In an informal study conducted shortly after opening the practice, 65 clients who experienced successful therapy outcomes were asked what was most helpful. As Lipchik (2014) stated: "Not one client ever credited a particular technique or homework task as having made a difference to them. Instead, they reported things like the therapist 'accepted me . . . understood what I was saying, and . . . made me feel better about myself'" (p. 71). These findings highlighted the role of the therapeutic relationship and client emotions in SFT, as she later described in the book *Beyond Technique in Solution-Focused Therapy: Working With Emotions and the Therapeutic Relationship* (Lipchik, 2002).

O'Hanlon and Weiner-Davis

With the 1989 publication of *In Search of Solutions,* Bill O'Hanlon and Michelle Weiner-Davis were among the first clinicians besides de Shazer to publish a book about solution-focused practice. Weiner-Davis had completed the formal training program at BFTC a few years before O'Hanlon invited her to collaborate on the book. A revised version was published in 2003 (O'Hanlon & Weiner-Davis, 2003), and both authors have published other books on solution-focused practice with struggling couples (Weiner-Davis, 1992), trauma (O'Hanlon & Bertolino, 2002), and other client challenges.

Dolan

Yvonne Dolan, a cofounder of the Solution-Focused Brief Therapy Association, has coauthored books with Berg and de Shazer that include *Tales of Solutions* (Berg & Dolan, 2001) and *More Than Miracles* (de Shazer et al., 2021). She also coauthored a book on the use of SFT in agency settings (Pichot & Dolan, 2003) and is considered an expert on SFT with people who have experienced sexual abuse (Dolan, 1991) and other traumas (Dolan, 2000).

Korman, Furman, and Macdonald

Psychiatrists Harry Korman from Sweden, Alasdair Macdonald from Great Britain, and Ben Furman from Finland have published extensively and taught SFT to thousands of practitioners in their respective countries and beyond. Korman coauthored *More Than Miracles* (de Shazer et al., 2021) and has conducted microanalyses on differences between client–therapist dialogue in SFT and other approaches (Korman et al., 2013). Among his most enduring contributions is an online solution-focused discussion group (https://www.sikt.nu/sft-l) he established in 1995 as a communication vehicle for the solution-focused community. Although he recently stepped down as list manager, the list remains the largest international forum for exchanging information and ideas on SFT practice, training, and research.

Ben Furman, a child/family psychiatrist in Helsinki, has written several books and conducted trainings in many different countries. His first book, *Solution Talk*, was cowritten with Tapani Ahola (Furman & Ahola, 1992), a social psychologist who has collaborated with Furman on various projects over the years. Furman has published on team building and self-help, and created the Kids Skills program (Furman, 2010) to help children resolve social, emotional, and behavioral problems in solution-focused ways. He has also developed solution-focused mental health apps for children and adults.

Alasdair Macdonald is an experienced clinician with a long list of publications that includes *Solution-Focused Therapy: Theory, Research and Practice*, now in its second edition (Macdonald, 2011). For many years, he posted a running list of SFT research studies called the evaluation list. The list is currently maintained by the European Brief Therapy Association and remains a popular resource among SFT practitioners, researchers, and trainers.

BRIEF

As word of SFT spread during the 1980s and 1990s, brief therapy centers were opened in various parts of the world to provide solution-focused clinical and training services. One of the earliest and most visible centers was BRIEF (short for BRIEF Centre for Solution-Focused Practice) in London, England. Founded in 1989 by Evan George, Chris Iveson, and Harvey Ratner, BRIEF's inaugural conference featured de Shazer and Berg. These therapists (who were joined by Guy Shennan from 2004 to

2010) resonated with the efficiency and parsimony of SFT and have further simplified and modified the approach over the years (Ratner et al., 2012). In addition to using fewer end-of-session messages and tasks as compared with BFTC, they shifted from talking about clients' goals, miracles, and exceptions—which they saw as unnecessarily tied to the client's problem—to talking about clients' best hopes, preferred futures, and instances of preferred futures. The BRIEF team has provided SFT classes and training workshops throughout Europe and beyond.

Researchers: Franklin, Kim, Beyebach, Bavelas, Smock Jordan, and De Jong

Research has played a significant role in SFT's growth and development starting with the Milwaukee group and continuing through the efforts of hundreds of others. The following researchers have made major contributions to the evidence base of SFT.

Cynthia Franklin, professor at the University of Texas at Austin, has published dozens of empirical studies over the past several decades. She served as lead editor of *Solution-Focused Brief Therapy: A Handbook of Evidence-Based Practice* and has written extensively on the application of SFT in schools (Franklin et al., 2018). Johnny Kim, a former student of Franklin, has followed his mentor's lead by serving as lead researcher on several meta-analyses (Kim et al., 2015, 2019), writing *Solution-Focused Brief Therapy: A Multicultural Approach* (Kim, 2014), and publishing other studies and works on the approach.

Mark Beyebach has conducted dozens of studies on the language of SFT as part of the brief therapy research program in Salamanca, Spain, beginning in 1989. Many of the studies are classified as process–outcome research that examine SFT processes and techniques and their relationship to client outcomes (Beyebach, 2014). He has recently investigated the global use and impact of SFT in different countries and cultures around the world, which has further confirmed SFT's status as a transculturally relevant and effective therapy approach (Beyebach et al., 2021; Neipp & Beyebach, 2022).

Janet Beavin Bavelas, who died in 2022, was an experimental psychologist, communications researcher at MRI and University of Victoria, and expert in microanalysis research and methodology. She spent the bulk of her career meticulously observing and documenting the details of human dialogue in therapy and other contexts. Bavelas took a special interest in the coconstructive nature of solution-focused dialogue and teamed up with others to examine differences between client–therapist interactions in SFT and other therapy approaches (Bavelas et al., 2014; Korman et al., 2013).

Two members of Bavelas's microanalysis research team—Sara Smock Jordan and Peter De Jong—have contributed to SFT research and clinical literature in many different ways. Smock Jordan, a founding member of the Solution-Focused Brief Therapy Association, has developed a solution-focused inventory (Smock et al., 2010), collaborated on two meta-analyses (Kim et al., 2010, 2019), and published dozens of other empirical and clinical articles on SFT. De Jong's empirical and clinical writings over the past three decades have clarified the process of SFT and reinforced its credibility and evidence base. In addition to his work on microanalysis and coconstruction in SFT (De Jong et al., 2013, 2020), he conducted the first systematic review of SFT outcome research (De Jong & Hopwood, 1996) and coauthored (with Berg) *Interviewing for Solutions,* now in its fourth edition (De Jong & Berg, 2013).

CONTEMPORARY SOLUTION-FOCUSED THERAPY

SFT cofounders de Shazer and Berg continued to refine and teach solution-focused practice up to the time of their deaths in 2005 and 2007, respectively. Although the BFTC closed its doors in 2007, the work at the center has inspired a new generation of practitioners and a growing number of developments, adaptations, applications, research studies, and writings on SFT—several of which are included in this book, such as developments and writings of BRIEF (Ratner et al., 2012), microanalyses (Bavelas et al., 2014), incorporation of systematic client feedback (Gillaspy & Murphy, 2012), and transcultural applications of SFT (Neipp & Beyebach, 2022).

The effectiveness of any therapy approach depends largely on its cultural relevance and responsiveness. Given that SFT is compatible with recommendations and best practices in multiculturalism and diversity-competent clinical practice (De Jong & Berg, 2013; D. W. Sue et al., 2019), it is not surprising that it has been effective with a diversity of clients in many different countries and cultures throughout of the world (Kim, 2014; Neipp & Beyebach, 2022). SFT has also been used in a variety of contexts such as coaching, business settings, community planning, schools, crisis hotlines, and others (McKergow, 2021). It has also proven successful with a wide range of client difficulties, including trauma (Froerer et al., 2018), substance misuse (Hendrick et al., 2012; Pichot & Smock, 2009), schizophrenia (Panayotov et al., 2012), self-harming (Selekman, 2009), suicide prevention (Fiske, 2017), and relationship problems, to name just a few. Last, the efficiency of SFT is well suited to clients' time constraints, financial/geographical restrictions, and other practical realities.

SUMMARY

Dissatisfied with the status quo of psychotherapy and inspired by the work of Erickson and MRI, de Shazer, Berg, and a small group of clinicians opened the BFTC of Milwaukee in 1978 to explore different ways to approach therapy. They recorded and examined hundreds of real-life therapy sessions with a focus on the practical question "What do therapist and clients talk about when therapy is successful?" The answers that emerged over the next decade formed the bases of an innovative approach called solution-focused therapy that challenged long-standing precepts and practices of psychotherapy.

Instead of diagnosing and exploring client problems, solution-focused therapists identified what clients wanted from therapy and what they already had toward achieving it. Although the BFTC closed its doors shortly after the deaths of de Shazer and Berg, the core ideas and methods of the Milwaukee group live on through thousands of contemporary SFT researchers, clinicians, and trainers. The following chapters describe the theory, process, and evaluation of this unique approach to psychotherapy.

3

Theory

. . . in solution building with clients, we never ask why.

—De Jong & Berg, 2013, p. 366

This chapter describes the goals, tenets, and additional theoretical features that distinguish solution-focused therapy (SFT) from other psychotherapy approaches. It also explains how theory itself has been conceptualized and developed in SFT, with emphasis on de Shazer's ideas and writings.

ROLE OF THEORY IN SFT

Although SFT has been misunderstood as lacking a theory, a careful review of writings on the approach confirms that theory has always been part of its development. For example, Korman et al. (2020) reported that at least one third of the content in de Shazer's writings (six books, 75 papers) pertained to theory. When de Shazer said SFT "had no theory," he was likely referring to the fact that solution-focused techniques were developed inductively by analyzing therapy videos and replicating or refining therapeutic interactions associated with client improvements—an approach better known today as "grounded theory" (Corbin & Strauss, 2015). This inductive approach distinguishes SFT from psychotherapies that were deduced and formulated from established theories of personality and psychopathology.

Theory With a Small "t"

The role of theory in SFT is unconventional when compared with other theories of psychotherapy. As reported by Korman et al. (2020), de Shazer differentiated between an uppercase-T *Theory* and lowercase-t *theory*—the former being general and global, the latter being specific and pragmatic. When de Shazer told people SFT had no theory, he was referring to theory in its uppercase sense, not in its more limited lowercase sense. The following quotes elaborate on this distinction and other ideas about the role and nature of theory in SFT.

> Theory, as I use the term, is not meant as an "explanation," [i.e., inferences] but rather as a coherent "description" of specific sequences of events within a specific context [i.e., a description of the therapist interacting with the client in the therapy setting]. (de Shazer, 1988, p. xiv)

> The theory has nothing whatsoever to say about "problems complaints, difficulties" etc. In fact, the theory explicitly neither includes nor excludes ideas about causation and neither includes nor excludes the various ideas about problem maintenance: it only deals with doing therapy. (de Shazer, 1988, p. xix)

> In order to construct a useful theory of doing (brief) therapy, we need to identify what is observable and repeatable about therapy sessions. We need to describe the consistencies from session to session and case to case based on what therapists and clients actually do during therapy sessions. Therefore, theory development needs to be based on the disciplined observation of therapy being done within a specific

context. From this process, a description of what is done in therapy sessions can be built and then rules can be created that will enable other people to do therapy "in the same way." (Gingerich & de Shazer, 1991, pp. 241–242)

These quotes highlight the unconventional nature of theory and theory construction in SFT. In a comprehensive review of SFT theory based on de Shazer's writings, Korman et al. (2020) noted the following differences in the construction and scope of solution-focused theory compared to other psychotherapy theories:

- Whereas theory construction in many approaches begins with propositions about the nature and cause of human problems, SFT does not theorize about client behaviors or problems outside of the observable client–therapist interactions in which they are described.
- The scope of SFT theory is considerably narrower than the scope of other psychotherapy theories.
- Theory construction and research in SFT focuses on the pragmatic question "What do therapists and clients talk about when therapy is successful?" The answers (descriptions) that have emerged from this question form the basis of SFT theory. For example, SFT theory proposes that having clients discuss what they want more of in their lives enhances therapy outcomes. There is no speculation as to why this is the case or how it works, only a description of what it looks like in a therapy session.
- The scope of SFT theory is limited to how change happens in the therapy context and nothing more. The theoretical value of such descriptions is that they can be replicated and refined across different therapists, clients, problems, cultures, and settings. As Korman et al. (2020) pointed out, generations of solution-focused therapists have drawn on these descriptions to assist clients in living more satisfying lives.

WITTGENSTEIN'S INFLUENCE

During the latter part of his career, de Shazer was influenced by the language-related ideas of philosopher Ludwig Wittgenstein. For example, he adopted Wittgenstein's (1953) preference for observation and description over conjecture and explanation and often cited Wittgenstein's belief that it was a mistake to seek an explanation for something when all one needed was a description of how it worked. This belief is evidenced in SFT's emphasis on eliciting meticulous descriptions of clients' preferred futures, exceptions, and progress toward desired outcomes.

de Shazer also appreciated Wittgenstein's ideas on the interactional and contextual quality of human language and meaning making, stating that "Wittgenstein . . . points out that the meaning of words is determined by how they are used by the various participants in a specific context" (de Shazer, 1991, p. 71) and that "language and speech originate and develop through use, through social interaction and communication" (de Shazer, 1994, p. 51). These ideas fit well with social constructionism's view of therapy as a coconstructive process in which new meanings are created through client–therapist dialogues (McNamee & Gergen, 1992). The coconstruction of new meanings and solutions is central to SFT theory and practice.

GOALS OF SFT

The main goal of SFT is to elicit detailed descriptions of the client's desired outcome and build on exceptions and resources that support the outcome. This goal translates into three main tasks (along with sample questions that address each task):

- Setting a direction ("What are your best hopes from this?" "What will be different when you achieve this?")
- Building on client exceptions and resources ("When was the problem less noticeable last week?" "How did you make that happen?" "What/who else might be helpful?")
- Exploring progress toward desired outcomes ("Where would you put yourself on the 0–10 scale?" "What's been better since our last meeting?")

Solution-focused questions and conversations reflect a shift from diagnosing and correcting what is wrong with clients to identifying and increasing what is right and working in their lives. Although solution-focused therapists may assign a diagnosis when clients request it, they typically collaborate with clients to arrive at a diagnosis—and do not discuss it further unless the client chooses to.[1]

Because SFT assumes that clients have the resources needed to improve their lives, the therapist's goal is to facilitate client-directed solutions. These solutions may have little or nothing to do with the problem that brought the client to therapy.

TENETS OF SFT

The following tenets guide the practice of SFT and distinguish it from other approaches (de Shazer et al., 2021; Korman et al., 2020; Murphy, 2023).

If It's Not Broken, Don't Fix It

SFT focuses on the stated concerns and goals of clients and nothing more. This immediately distinguishes it from approaches that assess and treat areas outside of the client's stated concern as determined by the therapist's judgment or theoretical model. As de Shazer et al. (2021) noted:

> Nothing would seem more absurd than to intervene upon a situation that is already resolved. While this seems obvious, in reality there are some schools of psychotherapy that would encourage therapy "for growth" . . . or to get to "deeper meanings" and structures. SFBT is antithetical to these. If there is no problem, there should be no therapy. (pp. 1–2)

---

[1] Clients rarely request a formal diagnosis unless they need it for insurance purposes. Solution-focused therapists do not routinely assign diagnoses to clients for the following reasons: (a) Diagnosis is a problem-focused process that lacks adequate validity and reliability; (b) diagnosis objectifies clients and disregards their complexity, multidimensionality, and resources; (c) diagnosis offers minimal direction on resolving problems; (d) diagnosis may compress clients' thinking, hope, and self-identities in ways that reduce solution options and possibilities; (e) diagnosis locates problems within clients and may exclude social/ecological solutions in favor of medication, individual therapy, or other internal/individual interventions; and (f) clients may "become" their diagnosis when they view it as fact versus construction. Refer to Murphy and Sparks (2018, pp. 41–44) for a longer discussion of diagnosis as it applies to SFT and other strengths-based approaches.

If It Works, Do More of It

This guideline captures the essence of SFT and the corresponding assumption that all clients bring useful resources to the therapy table—personal attributes, strengths, exceptions, social supports, and other indigenous resources that may help them achieve desired outcomes. Rather than trying to give clients something they do not already have, solution-focused therapists invite them to notice, describe, and expand on existing exceptions and resources. For example, when working with partners who want to enhance their relationship, the therapist might invite them to pay special attention to the times they get along a little better than usual, describe personal actions and resources associated with those times, and build on these actions and resources in the future.

If It Doesn't Work, Do Something Different

This seemingly obvious guideline is not as easy as it sounds. Human beings have the unique tendency to continually repeat an attempted solution despite its ineffectiveness in resolving the problem—especially when the solution is seen as the only sensible response to the problem. This guideline applies to clients and therapists alike. No matter how reasonable a strategy may seem to the therapist, its value rests entirely on how the client responds to it and benefits from it. Instead of calling clients resistant or otherwise faulting them when they do not respond to a particular question or technique, SFT clinicians try something different.

Imagine working with a parent who reports that their repeated attempts to "talk sense into" their child have not worked. Rather than attempting to analyze or explain why it hasn't worked, the solution-focused therapist might invite something different by saying, "I wonder what you might think of or do that's very different from anything you've tried so far." For many clients, SFT itself may represent "something different" from their previous efforts to improve the situation, including previous therapy experiences.

Clients Are Resourceful

Solution-focused therapists fully acknowledge the demoralizing impact of serious problems *and* the potential of all clients to deploy their strengths and resources toward solutions. This tenet is based on the idea that life requires an ample degree of resilience and capability and that clients are always managing and solving problems.

SFT also assumes that clients know what they want from therapy and, with the assistance of the therapist or other people in their lives, can effectively apply their resources toward desired outcomes. This does not imply that clients would not benefit from additional knowledge and skills or that therapists can resolve skill-based difficulties (e.g., reading or speech problems) by talking with clients in solution-focused ways. It simply means that SFT invites clients to build on what is already available and working in their lives—values, successes, motivations, relationships, resilience, creativity, and other existing resources.

SFT theory proposes that it is more respectful and expedient to build solutions from naturally occurring client exceptions and resources rather than relying solely on practitioner interventions. SFT clients are seen as stuck versus sick and problems are seen as roadblocks versus symptoms of internal pathology. This viewpoint boosts hope, expands solution opportunities, and centralizes the input and contributions of clients.

Clients Are Cooperative

In SFT, it is the therapist's job to cooperate with clients and not the other way around. This guideline applies to all clients, including those who enter therapy reluctantly at the urging of courts, parents, partners, or social service agencies. Instead of viewing clients as resistant and trying to coerce their cooperation, solution-focused therapists assume that clients are always cooperating in ways that make sense to them at the time. For example, suppose the therapist invites the client to consider talking with their supervisor about a problem they're having at work, and the client does not do so. Instead of confronting the client or assuming they were being lazy or resistant, the therapist would view it as useful communication that the timing, content, or other aspects of the invitation did not fit for the client. SFT practitioners also assume that every client will cooperate in working toward self-selected therapy goals that are important and meaningful to them.

Nothing Happens Constantly

This principle draws on the notion that all aspects of life, including problems, change and fluctuate over time. No matter how constant a problem may seem to those who experience it, there are always variations in its presence and intensity. These variations or exceptions are central to SFT theory and practice.

The fact that exceptions or instances of the client's preferred future are always happening to some extent has practical implications for what is discussed in therapy. In SFT, these events and experiences are core building blocks for solutions. More specifically, solution-focused therapists assist clients in identifying, exploring, and expanding the presence of exceptions in their lives. For example, when working with a struggling couple seeking to improve their relationship, the therapist would invite them to think of a recent time or situation when things were better than usual between them ("Tell me about a time this week when you got along a tad bit better than usual"). If the couple said their dinner conversation Tuesday evening was more pleasant than most of their recent dinners, then the therapist would explore relevant differences between Tuesday's conversation and other ones, including what each of them did differently to make it happen ("What did you do differently?"). Finally, the couple might be invited to be on the lookout for similar exceptions during the coming week.

Small Changes Can Lead to Big Changes

This tenet reflects SFT's systemic and pragmatic origins. Since solution construction often involves small steps toward a better future, solution-focused therapists are attentive to small changes throughout the therapy process. Noticing and exploring small changes is based on the systemic notion that one change leads to another, then another, and so on until the client views their situation as good enough for therapy to end. The idea that small changes may lead to bigger and more meaningful changes is a useful source of hope for clients and therapists.

This principle is illustrated with Leah, a successful bank officer who complained of depression and wanted to feel more enthusiastic. Early in the first session, the therapist asked Leah where she would put herself on a 0–10 scale of enthusiasm and where she needed to be to consider therapy successful enough to end. Leah said she was at a 3 and would need to be at a 7 to end therapy. At the end of the session, the therapist invited her to be on the lookout for the *first small sign* of movement toward a 3.1 on the scale. Leah began the second session by telling the therapist she had moved to a 5 on the scale, adding that the first small sign of progress was spending a couple of minutes in the evening selecting a work outfit for the next day. This was followed by waking up a little earlier than usual on two or three occasions. Leah described additional small signs of progress that accounted for her higher rating. She ended therapy two sessions later when she reached her good enough rating of 7. As seen with Leah and many clients, one or two small changes can lead to larger and more meaningful changes.

The Solution Is Not Necessarily Related to the Problem

In contrast to therapy approaches in which an adequate assessment and understanding of the problem is a necessary first step, SFT begins by inviting clients to describe how their lives would be different without the problem. This description guides the therapy process from that point on as clients and therapists identify exceptions or "times when portions of the desired solution description already exist or could potentially exist in the future" (de Shazer et al., 2021, p. 2).

Solution-focused practitioners listen to and validate the client's problem but do not gather detailed information about it. They are more interested in what clients want (vs. don't want) and what they have (vs. lack) toward achieving it. They help clients build solutions from naturally occurring successes, strengths, and other personal/social resources that may have nothing to do with the problem. The idea that the solution is not necessarily related to the problem represents a paradigm shift that distinguishes SFT from problem-focused approaches. Table 3.1 outlines other differences between problem-focused and solution-focused therapy.

The Language of Solutions Is Different From the Language of Problems

This tenet, like the previous one, reveals key differences between problem-focused and solution-focused language and conversations. Language is a major tool of therapy and solution-focused therapists are very intentional

Table 3.1

Differences Between Problem-Focused and Solution-Focused Therapy

Problem-focused therapy	Solution-focused therapy
What is lacking/flawed/unwanted?	What is available/working/wanted?
Causes of problem/complaint—why?	Paths to solution/preferred future—what/how?
Diagnose/detail/decrease problem	Identify/detail/increase exceptions
Interpretive	Descriptive
Problem-solving language	Solution-building language
Therapist-directed	Client-directed
Therapist is expert on client	Client is expert on self
Client cooperates with therapist	Therapist cooperates with client
Dialogue is backdrop of change	Dialogue is key means of change
Many assumptions about clients/solutions	Few assumptions about clients/solutions
Solutions are prescribed by therapist	Solutions are coconstructed with client
Medical model—client is sick/symptomatic	Strengths model—client is stuck/resourceful

Note. Adapted from *Solution-Focused Counseling in Schools* (4th ed., p. 48), by J. J. Murphy, 2023, American Counseling Association. Copyright 2023 by American Counseling Association. Adapted with permission.

in their use of it. As Berg and de Shazer (1993) noted, "Our clients have taught us that solutions involve a very different kind of thinking and talking . . . that is . . . outside the problem" (p. 9). Whereas problem talk tends to focus on the past and the permanence of problems, solution talk tends to be future-focused, suggestive of the problem's transience, and centered on the aspects of clients and their lives that support their goals. Solution-focused therapists respectfully acknowledge the pain of the problem while inviting clients to describe what they want instead. The yes–and interplay between acknowledging problems and constructing solutions conveys empathy for the client's current struggle ("*Yes*, you are in a very tough spot now . . .") and curiosity about their hoped-for future (". . . *and* I'm wondering what you want to be different in the future"). These conversations invite people to shift from talking themselves into problems to talking themselves out of them.

The usefulness of solution talk is supported by social construction-ism theory (Gergen, 2015) and detailed microanalyses of the content and impact of client–therapist language and dialogue (Bavelas et al., 2014). In a microanalysis of 120 therapy sessions, therapists who spent more time discussing client strengths and resources were more successful than those who talked more about client problems (Gassmann & Grawe, 2006). The investigators concluded that clients benefit from experiencing themselves as more than the sum of their problems. Microanalyses have also confirmed that solution-focused therapists were more likely to dis-cuss positive features of clients' lives than cognitive behavior therapy prac-titioners (Froerer & Jordan, 2013; Smock Jordan et al., 2013) and that SFT sessions included more positive content from therapists *and* clients than cognitive behavior therapy and motivational interviewing sessions (Korman et al., 2013; Smock Jordan et al., 2013). These findings support SFT's emphasis on the purposeful use of language, the coconstructive power of solution-focused dialogue, and the notion that the more time one spends talking about something the more salient and meaningful it becomes in one's thinking and life.

As a result of their family therapy backgrounds and MRI training, de Shazer and Berg were influenced by *systems theory* when they began to develop the solution-focused approach in Milwaukee. As the approach evolved, *social constructionism* became a more central framework for guiding and conceptualizing what happens in SFT. These influences are examined below along with their practical implications and benefits.

SYSTEMS THEORY

Solution-focused therapists view clients, problems, and solutions from an interactional or systemic perspective based on the following assumptions from systems theory: (a) Clients exist in social systems such as families, communities, societies, and other systems; (b) social interactions strongly influence the way clients see themselves, others, and the world; (c) the problems that bring clients to therapy are embedded in social contexts versus residing strictly within the client; and (d) a small change in one part of the system can lead to bigger changes in other parts. The practical benefits of approaching clients and therapy from a systemic perspective are described below.

The systemic perspective of SFT creates *more flexibility and solution-building options* compared to an individualistic perspective that situates problems inside the client and views symptoms as signs of internal pathology. For example, a systemic perspective encourages solution-building options beyond the individual client such as involving significant others, making environmental changes, and so forth.

The systemic idea that *small changes can lead to bigger changes* encourages therapists and clients to be watchful for small indications of hope and progress whenever or wherever they may occur. For example, SFT practitioners frequently invite clients to be on the lookout for small signs of exceptions and progress that occur between sessions.

The systemic perspective of SFT has also prompted *additional therapeutic techniques* that address key relationships and social interactions in the client's life. For example, "relationship questions" invite clients to describe the details and significance of social relationships, interactions, and events associated with desired outcomes, exceptions, and progress ("What will your partner notice as you become more relaxed?" "What did she do when you held it together instead of losing it?" "How is your relationship different now compared to when we started meeting?").

Another advantage of SFT's systemic perspective is that it *promotes hope and reduces blame* by focusing on small changes and solution opportunities beyond the individual client. The more pathways there are to desired outcomes, the more hope clients will have toward achieving them. Another benefit of systemic thinking is that it reduces the likelihood of blaming clients for the problems they experience. Blame tends to impede clients' resourcefulness and flexibility at the very time they need it most. Adopting a systemic view of problems and solutions counteracts the tendency to blame clients and encourages a more compassionate, collaborative, multifaceted approach to building solutions.

SOCIAL CONSTRUCTIONISM

The tenets and techniques of SFT are supported by the following propositions of social constructionism theory (Gergen, 2015):

- People's sense of what is real is personally constructed rather than discovered through purely objective means.
- Personal constructions result largely from social interactions, language, and dialogue.
- These internalized constructions strongly influence (for better or worse) one's self-perceptions, actions, and hopes.

From a social constructionist standpoint, diagnoses and other "professional" ideas and theories are just that—ideas and theories constructed by people rather than objective truths about the client or problem. Although these theories are constructions versus facts, their impact is very real. As Shapiro et al. (2006) noted, personal constructions "affect the individual's self-concept, . . . understanding of her past, . . . and behavior in the future, because we behave in accordance with what we believe to be possible" (pp. 137–138).

The impact of language and dialogue on personal constructions speaks to the coconstructive potential therapeutic conversations have in changing the way clients view themselves and their capabilities. In a microanalysis of 120 sessions involving 30 clients and 23 therapists, Gassmann and Grawe (2006) reported that the least successful therapists spent more time discussing clients' problems, while the most successful ones spent more time discussing clients' strengths and resources. The authors concluded that clients need to experience themselves as more than the sum of their problems. These findings support SFT's emphasis on the purposeful use of words and language, coconstructive power of dialogue, and other positive effects of solution talk—all of which contribute to an increasingly hopeful and progressive client story.

This coconstructive process of SFT, sometimes called *solution building* (De Jong & Berg, 2013), involves listening, selecting, and building. The therapist *listens* for and *selects* key client words and phrases, then *builds* subsequent questions or comments from what the client has said. For example, when a client in couples therapy says, "We're not as comfortable with each other as we used to be," the therapist might say, "Tell me about a recent time you were a bit more comfortable with each other." The ongoing process of listening, selecting, and building on the client's natural language enables therapists and clients to coconstruct new meanings and possibilities. The coconstructive process of SFT has been validated in studies that report the positive impact of solution-focused questions and conversations on clients' emotions, self-efficacy, and actions (Grant, 2012; Neipp et al., 2016; Zhai & Zhu, 2016).

CULTURAL CONSIDERATIONS

This section describes how SFT theory aligns with research and best practices in multicultural counseling and therapy, with emphasis on the benefits of adopting a multicultural orientation. A multicultural orientation refers to how a therapist views and values cultural diversity, which affects the way they work with clients from all backgrounds and intersectional identities (Hook et al., 2017). Adopting a multicultural orientation requires therapists to (a) acknowledge that they can never fully understand a client's cultural experience, and (b) incorporate elements of clients' cultural backgrounds and everyday lives that can help them achieve desired outcomes. As discussed shortly, cultural humility and responsiveness are cornerstones of a multicultural orientation.

Inviting clients to apply their indigenous strengths and resources toward therapeutic goals is central to SFT, as is the therapist's awareness of potentially adverse effects that certain sociocultural messages, injustices, and experiences may have on clients. Although this point applies to all clients, it is particularly relevant to persons from underrepresented groups that include people of color, clients living in poverty, persons of nondominant sexual orientations, and clients with developmental disabilities, to name a few.

There are many challenges to providing culturally responsive services, beginning with the fact that most therapists are from dominant groups. For example, most mental health practitioners come from White, middle-class backgrounds that promote Western values such as individualism, self-reliance, and autonomy (Ivey et al., 2018). Although these values might work well for some clients, they may miss the mark for underrepresented clients who have experienced systemic racism, discrimination, and other contextual influences that adversely affect them. These concerns may partly explain why traditional therapy approaches have been largely unsuccessful with clients from nondominant groups (S. Sue & Zane, 2006)—and why obtaining and accommodating client feedback are essential elements of culturally responsive services (Murphy & Sparks, 2018).

Unfortunately, the well-intentioned efforts to improve therapists' multicultural effectiveness may inadvertently perpetuate the very problems they seek to resolve. For example, some forms of "cultural competency" training have required people to memorize specific customs and traits of different cultural groups. While this type of training may help expand one's overall knowledge of cultural diversity and differences, it can undermine the complexity of people and reinforce the stereotyped notion that all clients from a particular racial or ethnic group share similar characteristics. It may also minimize the intersectionality of a client's diverse identities (parent, person of color, cisgender partner, employee, friend, etc.) and their relative importance in the client's life (Price et al., 2019). Finally, traditional cultural competency training has been criticized for (a) implying that therapists can achieve cultural competency through intellectual knowledge and awareness, (b) focusing on client-related cultural factors with minimal attention to therapist factors and client–therapist power disparities, and (c) implying (through the word "competency") that it is possible for a therapist to become fully competent in culture-related knowledge and skills (Hook et al., 2017).

For reasons noted above, cultural competency is an outdated concept that has been replaced by *cultural responsiveness* and *cultural humility* (Hook et al., 2017). Both terms capture the dynamic process of accommodating and adapting to the limitless perspectives and identities of clients. Cultural humility is embodied in the attitude and actions of solution-focused therapists. For example, solution-focused therapists approach every client with a fresh sense of curiosity and openness—along with a willingness to learn from clients and adjust services based on their preferences and perspectives versus those of the therapist, therapy model, or larger society.

Cultural humility requires therapists to approach every client as a culture of one and every session as a cross-cultural exchange (Murphy & Sparks, 2018). This enables solution-focused therapists to avoid stereotyping clients on the basis of diagnostic categories, prior experiences with similar clients, or anything else that diminishes the uniqueness and complexity of the person in front of them. These ideas and methods are advocated by multicultural researchers and theorists who consistently recommend giving clients a central voice in establishing therapy goals, evaluating the effectiveness of services, and other key aspects of their care (D. W. Sue et al., 2019). SFT practitioners apply these recommendations by centralizing the input and contributions of clients in all aspects of their care. Although cultural humility and responsiveness involve approaching clients from a position of not knowing, this does not imply passivity on the therapist's part when it comes to increasing one's multicultural knowledge and skills and one's knowledge and awareness of personal biases— an active and ongoing process for therapists of all theoretical orientations.

Building on clients' indigenous strengths and resources is another way in which SFT promotes culturally responsive services for all clients (D. W. Sue et al., 2019). As Ridley (2005) noted, "While vigorously looking for psychopathology in . . . minority clients, therapists often miss opportunities to help clients identify their assets and use these assets advantageously" (p. 103). Boyd-Franklin et al. (2013) similarly encouraged therapists to adopt a strengths-based approach with African American clients who may be more aware of their problems than their strengths. This is typically true for most clients regardless of their race, ethnicity, or cultural background.

Corey (2023) and Kim (2014) have observed that SFT is particularly well suited to working with clients from culturally underrepresented and underserved populations because the client's goal drives the therapy process; therapy centers on the client's language and preferences versus the therapist's language, preferences, and theories; and therapeutic solutions emerge from the client's strengths and resources rather than the therapist's interventions.

SUMMARY

Chapter 3 has examined the theory of SFT with attention to the main goals, tenets, and other theoretical features that inform its use and distinguish it from other approaches. Whereas other theories were deduced from global theories of personality and psychopathology, SFT theory was constructed primarily from observations of real-life therapy sessions and evidence-based answers to the question "What do therapists and clients talk about when therapy is successful?" As a result, the scope of SFT theory is narrowly focused on client–therapist interactions within the therapy context.

The theory of SFT is compatible with the language-related philosophy and ideas of Wittgenstein and social constructionism, especially the postmodern notion that therapy is a coconstructive process in which new meanings and possibilities are created through client–therapist language and dialogue. SFT theory is also supported by multicultural research and best practices literature highlighting the therapeutic benefits of centralizing clients' goals, perceptions, preferences, and resources. Chapter 4 describes the nuts and bolts of putting this "simple but not easy" approach into action.

4

The Therapy Process

We need practitioners to realize that much of the best work they do is
amplifying the strengths rather than repairing patient's weaknesses.
—Martin E. P. Seligman, APA Presidential Address (1998)

This chapter describes the solution-focused therapy (SFT) process by examining the role of the client, therapist, and client–therapist relationship; core tasks and techniques; and session structure. Two extended client illustrations are provided—one involving a 38-year-old Latinx client with stress and parenting concerns (Rosa), the other involving a 27-year-old African American client with a history of trauma, social anxiety, and homelessness (Jalen).[1]

---

[1] The names of clients in this chapter and certain details of their lives have been changed for confidentiality purposes. Transcripts of dialogue were largely unaltered unless the client said something that could identify them and compromise confidentiality.

https://doi.org/10.1037/0000370-004
Solution-Focused Therapy, by J. J. Murphy

ROLE OF THE THERAPIST, CLIENT, AND CLIENT–THERAPIST RELATIONSHIP

The following discussion describes the active partnership and roles of solution-focused therapists and clients.

Role of the Therapist

According to de Shazer et al. (2021), the role of the therapist in SFT "tends to be more egalitarian and democratic than authoritarian" (pp. 3–4). In contrast to authoritarian approaches in which clinicians prescribe solutions based on their professional expertise and theory, solution-focused therapists elicit solutions from clients by approaching them from a stance of cultural humility (Hook et al., 2017), not knowing (H. Anderson, 2007), respectful curiosity (Murphy & Sparks, 2018), and leading from one step behind (Cantwell & Holmes, 1994). This stance is empirically supported by research on multicultural therapy, which has linked positive client outcomes to therapists' cultural humility (Davis et al., 2018; Hook et al., 2013). Adopting a stance of humility and not knowing is also supported by research findings linking successful client outcomes to healthy levels of therapist self-doubt (Nissen-Lie et al., 2017) and flexibility.

Solution-focused therapists lead the session but do so with gentle encouragement and "taps on the shoulder" of the client (Berg & Dolan, 2001, p. 3). This requires therapist humility and trust in clients' ability to improve their lives in the face of significant challenges. These features of the therapist's role convey the following message to the client: *You know yourself and your situation better than I do, so I will need your help in making our conversations as useful as possible for you.*

The role of the solution-focused therapist is similar to that of a foreign ambassador entering an unfamiliar country or culture (Murphy, 2023). Instead of beginning with preestablished ideas or recommendations, successful ambassadors (and therapists) ask clients what *they* want and encourage them to apply local resources toward achieving it. de Shazer et al. (2021) added that solution-focused therapists "almost never pass judgments about their clients, and avoid making any interpretations about the meanings behind their wants, needs, or behaviors" (p. 4). These attitudes and actions serve to centralize the client, decentralize the therapist, and promote the type of client participation and collaboration associated with successful outcomes (Tryon et al., 2019).

Role of the Client

Asking questions is central to solution-focused practice, so it is no surprise that answering questions and acting on their desired outcomes are the primary roles of clients in SFT. It's as simple as that, but a few aspects of this role warrant additional discussion. First, SFT assumes that the most effective solutions or "ways forward" come from clients rather than therapists. Second, it is assumed that talking with clients about their preferred future and related resources is the most efficient path to positive outcomes. This involves eliciting detailed descriptions of the client's preferred future that include personal, social, cognitive, and affective features—along with similar descriptions of exceptions, resources, and progress toward desired outcomes.

Language is important in any therapy approach, and SFT practitioners are especially mindful of their language and clients' language. That does not mean clients need to be verbose or eloquent speakers to benefit from SFT. It is difficult for clients to immediately provide the level of detail solution-focused therapists seek without struggling to some extent. These struggles tend to occur in early stages of the work, perhaps because the questions are different from what clients are expecting when they enter therapy. Since no two clients are alike, solution-focused therapists adapt their questions and conversations to the ability, style, and preferences of each client.

The accommodating nature of SFT is captured by the notion that the therapist works for the client, not the other way around. This does not mean that the role of the client is easy. Solution-focused questions are hard to answer, and therapists often stay with a question or topic for as long as it takes to elicit a sufficiently clear and detailed description. The coconstruction of concrete descriptions requires considerable persistence, patience, and hard work from therapists and clients alike. This is one reason solution-focused practice is considered "simple but not easy"— a phrase that aptly describes the client's role in SFT.

Role of the Client–Therapist Relationship

The client's experience of the client–therapist relationship or alliance has been consistently shown to affect therapy outcomes (Norcross & Lambert, 2019). The preceding discussion of therapist and client roles provides several hints about the role and nature of client–therapist relationships in SFT. Because solution-focused therapists view clients as experts on themselves, the alliance in SFT is "client directed" and driven by client hopes, perceptions, resources, and feedback. Solution-focused techniques are adapted to fit each client's personal style and preferences. These features of SFT mirror several core elements of evidence-based psychotherapy relationships (Norcross & Lambert, 2019).

Several aspects of SFT theory and practice enhance the establishment of strong alliances. For example, solution-focused therapists assume clients are always cooperating in ways that make sense to them and are motivated to work toward goals that matter to them. The therapist's job is to identify the client's desired outcome and ensure that all subsequent questions and conversations are linked to this outcome. When clients are not progressing, they are neither blamed nor deemed resistant. Instead, the therapist asks the client (a) how therapy sessions can be altered to make them more useful, (b) if their goal is still important to them, and (c) other questions aimed at becoming unstuck and moving forward.

Many SFT practitioners assume that positive client–therapist alliances will develop naturally as a result of the collaborative nature of solution-focused practice (Shennan, 2019). Others use two ultra-brief client feedback tools—the Outcome Rating Scale (ORS; Miller & Duncan, 2000) and the Session Rating Scale (SRS; Miller et al., 2002)—to obtain ongoing client perceptions of progress and the therapeutic alliance, respectively.[2] These scales are described and displayed in Appendix C, and their use in SFT is illustrated later in the client example involving Jalen.

The collaborative, client-directed alliance is evident in every phase of SFT from setting a direction at the start of therapy through deciding when to end services. Like other elements of SFT, the alliance centralizes clients and gives them a prominent voice in their care. This alliance is expressed in the core tasks and techniques of SFT.

CORE TASKS

The three main tasks of SFT are setting a direction, building on exceptions and other resources, and exploring progress. These interrelated tasks represent the entirety of solution-focused practice and occur in varying degrees and sequences in most sessions.

Task 1: Setting a Direction

Setting a direction is typically a two-step process that involves (a) eliciting the client's *desired outcome* from therapy (a generally stated hope or desired result from therapy), and (b) eliciting the client's *preferred future* (a specific, detailed, wide-ranging description of the desired outcome).

Eliciting the Client's Desired Outcome

The first step of setting a direction is to identify the client's desired outcome (also called *hoped-for outcome* or *goal*). SFT therapists do this in one of two ways, or a combination of both. First, they can use the ORS. The second and more commonly used option is to ask one of these questions: "What are your best hopes from therapy?" "If this turns out to be useful, what would be different to tell you it was useful?" or "How would you know coming here was not a waste of time?"

---

[2] The ORS and SRS are part of the evidence-based Partners for Change Outcome Management System (Duncan & Sparks, 2018). Although they are not considered standard features of SFT, some solution-focused therapists have encouraged their use because they are research-supported and consistent with SFT's client-centered emphasis (De Jong & Berg, 2013; Gillaspy & Murphy, 2012; Trepper & Franklin, 2012). See Appendix C for more information.

Regardless of which option is used, the therapist tries to elicit a broad and generally stated outcome. Since this is the first of two steps in setting a direction, general outcomes ("I'll be more relaxed around people") are favored over specific ones ("I'll talk with five people at the next office party") because overly specific goals limit the range of details and solutions that may emerge (during the second step of setting a direction) when the client and therapist coconstruct a detailed, wide-ranging description of the desired outcome referred to as the client's preferred future. A workable desired outcome and starting point for therapy may refer to the client's personal qualities or feelings (I'll be happier), key relationships (My partner and I will get along better), thinking (I'll be more focused at work), or anything else the client wants to do better or more of (being a better parent, managing my temper).

It is useful to think of the desired outcome as a client–therapist "contract" that drives the SFT process from that point on (Korman, 2004; Ratner et al., 2012). The outcome can be renegotiated as needed based on changes in clients' circumstances and preferences. As Korman (2004) noted, the desired outcome should be important to the client, achievable by the client and the therapy process, and within the therapist's ethical and legitimate scope of practice. As noted earlier, it should also be general enough to allow for a wide range of client descriptions and actions.

The following example involves Rosa, a 36-year-old Latinx woman who lived with her husband, Sal, and three children. Rosa sought therapy because of a growing sense of stress and anxiety, much of which involved concerns about her 7-year-old daughter Mia's "hyperactivity" and Rosa's confidence and ability as a parent. These concerns were affecting Rosa's ability to concentrate and be the parent she wanted to be for Mia and her other two children. The following dialogue is adapted from Murphy (2023, pp. 127–128) and begins about 5 minutes into the first session.

Therapist: What are your best hopes from talking with me?

Rosa: (*Pauses for several seconds*) I want to make sure I'm not part of the problem, you know, by how I respond to Mia. Sal is more patient than I am. I just want to be less uptight, you know, less tense when I'm dealing with Mia and my other kids.

Therapist: How do you want to be instead?

Rosa: Hmm. I'm not sure, but something needs to change with Mia, and I don't want to be part of the problem like I've read about in parent magazines. And I want Mia to do well in school because I know how important the first few years of school are. You know, they kind of set the tone for later.

Therapist: That make sense, and Mia is lucky to have you in her corner trying to make things better for her. [Acknowledging Rosa's efforts on Mia's behalf may help to counteract her discouragement and boost her confidence.]

Rosa: Well, thanks, but I'm worried about her. She's smart but easily distracted, and I'm not sure I'm helping, which stresses me out even more. We thought about medication, but that scares me a little because she's so young and I've heard about the side effects of some of those drugs. She's doing okay in school now, but things will be harder next year. I've read about ADHD kids and what parents should do to help them, but I have to constantly remind myself to do these things with Mia. Sometimes I just react in the moment, which usually ends up making things worse. That's why I want to talk things out with you, you know?

Therapist: Yes, that makes sense [validating Rosa's perceptions and concerns]. So, if talking things out with me ends up being useful, what will you be noticing to tell you it was useful? [The therapist echoes Rosa's process-based hope that "talking things out" will help, and then asks a question ("what will you be noticing . . . ?") aimed at eliciting an outcome that would enhance her everyday life "outside" of the therapy room.]

Rosa: Hmm. Do you mean with me or with Mia?

Therapist: Either you or Mia or both of you. And anything else you would notice to tell you it was helpful to talk things out here.

Rosa: I'd definitely be more chill, you know, and more patient with Mia and my other kids. Especially in the mornings when we're getting ready for work and getting them off to school and day care, all at the same time. It can be pretty chaotic.

Therapist: I'll bet it can. No wonder it's hard to be chill [validating Rosa's struggle].

Rosa: (*laughs*) Yes. My husband is more of a morning person, so he can handle the chaos better than I can.

Therapist: Okay, so, you would notice yourself being a little more chill or, uh, calmer and more patient in the morning. Is that it?

Rosa: Yes.

Therapist: So, if this ends up helping you become more chill and patient, what difference will that make in your life?

Rosa: (*pauses*) I'd be a better parent to Mia and my other kids.

In a matter of minutes and with the help of a few questions, Rosa was able to identify a desired outcome (being "more chill and patient" with her kids) that was achievable and broad enough to permit additional detailing and amplifying during the next step of setting a direction.

Eliciting the Client's Preferred Future

After eliciting the client's desired outcome (the first step of setting a direction), the therapist elicits a description of details and differences the client would notice should they achieve the outcome (the second step of setting a direction). This description is called the client's *preferred future* or *solution description*.

The Miracle Question. The most common way SFT practitioners elicit the client's preferred future is by asking the miracle question or similar questions. The *miracle question* was originally worded as follows: "Suppose that one night, while you were asleep, there was a miracle and this problem was solved. How would you know? What would be different? How will your husband know without your saying a word to him about it?" (de Shazer, 1988, p. 5). Of course, "husband" could be replaced with partner, friend, or other key persons in the client's life.

The versatility and effectiveness of this question led the Milwaukee group to begin using it with every client. As de Shazer (1988) noted:

"A framework for a whole series of questions (known collectively as 'the miracle question') is used in almost every first session . . . to help client and therapist alike to describe what a solution will look like" (p. 5). Clients became more hopeful as they described what postmiracle life would look like and be like for them. Because it was a client-produced description, it was seen by clients as possible and worthy of their best efforts.

The wording and delivery of the miracle question have been adapted to increase its effectiveness for a wide range of clients. For example, de Shazer et al. (2021) recommended asking the miracle question in a slow, deliberate, dramatic manner and occasionally pausing to help clients fully absorb the question and envision what postmiracle life would look like for them:

> Now, I want to ask you a strange question. Suppose that while you are sleeping tonight and the entire house is quiet, a miracle happens. The miracle is that the problem that brought you here is solved. However, because you are sleeping, you don't know that the miracle has happened. So, when you wake up tomorrow morning, what will be different to tell you a miracle has happened and the problem that brought you here is solved? (p. 5)

The miracle question can also be modified in various ways to fit the client's abilities, perspectives, and circumstances. For example, with clients who have experienced trauma and adamantly assert that they cannot forget or change the past, the miracle can be depicted as "unable to change the past but able to keep it from meddling with your future." When working with children, the question can be shortened ("If this problem disappeared just like that, how would things be different?"), supplemented by concrete/visual images ("imagine waving a special wand . . ."), and adapted in other ways that fit the developmental abilities and preferences of children (Murphy, 2023).

Similar Questions. Although the miracle question has received more attention in SFT research and literature than other methods of eliciting solution descriptions, any question that invites clients to describe hoped-for differences can do the job. Here are a few examples:

- If you woke up tomorrow and your hope of "being more relaxed" (client's desired outcome) was happening just as you wanted it to, what is the first thing you would notice? This "tomorrow question" was designed as an alternative to the miracle question because it does not refer to the client's problem (Ratner et al., 2012).

- Imagine it's 3 months from now and your life is where you want it to be. What would you be noticing to tell you things were different and better?
- What would be the first sign or two that you're more relaxed?
- How will you know the problem was solved?
- What will you/others be noticing to tell you/them that you no longer need therapy?

Most clients expect to be asked about their problems, so it is understandable when they struggle to answer questions about their best hopes and preferred futures—just as Rosa did when asked what she wanted instead of feeling stressed. However, with the help of the therapist's patience and gentle persistence, most clients can answer these questions. The following conversation about Rosa's preferred future picks up where the last one left off, just after she expressed her hope of being "more chill and patient."

Therapist: I have kind of a strange question for you. Imagine leaving here and going through the rest of the day and evening pretty much like any other day, okay? (*Rosa nods "yes."*) Then you go to bed and fall asleep. Sometime during the night, while you're sleeping, a miracle happens. (*pauses*) The miracle is that the problems that brought you here vanish, just like that (*snaps fingers*). But you don't know the miracle has happened because you were sleeping. What would be the very first thing you would notice the next morning to tell you the miracle happened?

Rosa: (*pauses*) Well, for starters, my kids wouldn't be screaming and fighting with each other about silly stuff, telling me what the other one did, stuff like that.

Therapist: What would you notice instead of the screaming and fighting? [When Rosa described what she didn't want, the therapist invited her to describe what she wanted instead. "Instead" questions invite a shift from problem talk to solution talk.]

Rosa: The kids would be playing and interacting in a positive way, you know, happy play. And I would wake up with more positive energy and feel more refreshed and rested. I'd probably find positive ways to be with Mia. Like I would get to enjoy her and enjoy her company instead of having to, you know, problem solve and break up skirmishes between her and her sisters and use all my energy for discipline. I'd be able to use my energy in a more positive way like playing, interacting, those sorts of things.

Therapist: What else would you be noticing?

Rosa: I'd feel more productive. I'd feel a sense of pride. I'd feel competent as a parent, like I was doing a good job. Feeling like my child is heading in a good direction, that sort of thing.

Therapist: Uh-huh.

Rosa: The biggest thing is probably feeling like I have the time and energy to give Mia more of the positive attention that she wants. Like playing a game with her, doing fun crafts and things like that. I think I would have the energy to do those things.

Therapist: What else would tell you you're on your way to becoming more patient?

Notice how the therapist followed up on Rosa's initial response to the miracle question with "What else?" questions to elicit a progressively wider and deeper description of her preferred future. As de Shazer et al. (2021) noted, effective preferred futures include "as many concrete details as possible" and clients' "emotions, thoughts, behaviors, and interactions with other people" (p. 52). The *3-S guideline* (Murphy, 2023) refers to three key features of effective preferred futures; 3-S stands for start based, specific, and social.

- **Start based:** Stated in positive terms as the start or presence of something the client wants versus the absence or reduction of what they don't want—for example, "waking up earlier" and "being on time for appointments" versus "being less depressed." When asked to describe what they want from therapy, many clients talk about what they do not want. When this occurs, the therapist asks what they want instead ("What would you rather be doing instead of being depressed?").

- **Specific:** In contrast to the client's generally stated desired outcome, the client's preferred future should be as specific, detailed, and wide-ranging as possible. Examples include "talking with mother once a week," "talking a walk after dinner," and "washing dishes before going to bed." No detail is too small or too specific when it comes to eliciting the client's preferred future. For example, one client responded to the miracle question by saying they would notice the pleasing scent of their hair after shampooing. The more specific the description, the more real and achievable it is for the client.

- **Social:** Addressing what significant others would notice, how they might respond, and what that would be like for the client—for example, "How will your family know you're more relaxed?" "What will they do?" "What will that be like for you?" Inviting clients to envision and describe how key people in their lives will react to desired changes can be an enlightening and motivating experience for them.

The start-based and specific features of effective preferred futures were evident in the previous dialogue with Rosa. As the conversation continued, the therapist explored social features by asking Rosa how her family might react to her positive changes. In addition to eliciting an increasingly detailed and multifaceted preferred future, these questions invited Rosa to discuss outward signs that would result from her feeling more patient and energetic following the miracle. Here are a few of her comments, many of which followed "What else?" questions from the therapist:

- Julia [Mia's little sister] would be happier. Even though they fight sometimes, Julia looks up to Mia and Mia usually enjoys helping her. So, I think we'd see a positive change in Julia, too, because she'd be getting attention from her big sister.
- Sal would be doing some of the same things I would, like having more positive interactions and less yelling and barking orders to the kids.
- It would be nice to be able to show attention to Julia without Mia getting jealous and trying to interject something to get attention for herself, which she does a lot.

- I would be able to parent my kids the way I want to, being positive and giving them the attention I want to give them.
- There would just be less stress in the air, you know. We'd all be more pleasant to each other.
- I'd have the time and energy to put into things I enjoy doing, and things my husband and I like doing together, like hiking. I can't think of the last time we went on a hike. Even something like cleaning the house, as weird as that may sound. Cleaning the house makes me feel better, more organized and on top of things. I like it when it's clean. So, if I had more cooperation from the kids, then they could even help around the house, which would be great. And there would be more time for me to just relax now and then. Really, for all of us to relax more.

At this point in the process, solution-focused therapists often ask clients to rate (on a 0–10 scale) where they are in relation to their preferred future and where they hope to be by the end of therapy. Rosa told the therapist she was at a 3 and needed to be at a 7 or 8 to end therapy. The client's preferred future description and scale ratings serve as reference points in subsequent conversations.

Setting a direction is the first and most important task of SFT because it guides everything that follows. Although setting a direction does not guarantee success, starting the work without a clear destination almost always guarantees failure.

Task 2: Building on Exceptions and Other Resources

Once a direction has been established, therapists invite clients to build on what is already in place in their lives to help them achieve desired outcomes. This involves building on exceptions as well as other client resources that are often discovered while exploring exceptions, preferred futures, and progress.

Exceptions refer to times, events, or situations in which the problem is absent or less noticeable, or times when the problem could have happened but did not. For a client who complains of debilitating social anxiety, exceptions might include recent social situations in which they were a little more relaxed than usual. Exceptions can also be seen as instances of the client's miracle description/preferred future (de Shazer et al., 2021). In this book, "exceptions" includes all of these situations and meanings. However, some solution-focused therapists prefer "instances" to exceptions because exceptions have historically been tied to the client's problem (Ratner et al., 2012).

Rationale for Building on Exceptions

Building on exceptions is based on the practical idea that it is more efficient to increase existing successes—no matter how small or infrequent—than it is to eliminate problems. The practicality of this strategy fits people's preference for simple versus complex solutions and for working *toward* something wanted versus away from something unwanted; as de Shazer (1987) observed, "if you want to go from point A to point B, but know no details of the terrain in between, the best thing to do is to assume that you can get from A to B by following a straight line" (p. 60). Increasing the frequency of exceptions is the straightest line from a problem to a solution.

Additional benefits of building on exceptions include the following: It is a versatile strategy applicable to every problem and every client; it has good "face validity" in that it makes sense to clients and is easy to understand; exceptions emerge from clients' everyday lives with no special intervention from the therapist (an empowering realization for clients who enter therapy down on themselves and discouraged by their difficulties); and clients become more hopeful and energized when they realize they are doing "something right" amidst their concerns and struggles— a useful consideration given the proven impact of hope on therapy outcomes (Hubble et al., 2010; Norcross & Lambert, 2019).

Process of Building on Exceptions

The 3-E process (Murphy, 2023) of building on exceptions involves *eliciting* exceptions, *exploring* the client's contributions and other exception-related details (e.g., when, where, how), and *expanding* the presence and magnitude of exceptions in the client's life. The first step is to elicit or find exceptions. In addition to asking questions, solution-focused therapists are always looking and listening for exceptions. For example, hints of exceptions may be found in psychological reports and other client records. Solution-focused therapists are also attentive to real time exceptions that occur during therapy sessions. Clients will often say or do something in a session that represents an exception. For example, a couple who wants to improve their relationship may display moments of empathy and compassion during a session. As small or fleeting as these exceptions may seem, they provide factual evidence of the couple's ability to achieve their desired outcome.

Therapists can also find hints of exceptions in the client's language. The italicized words in the following client comments provide hints of exceptions that can be further explored and detailed: "*Most* of my relationships have been awful," "I'm *almost always* late to work," "I *rarely* feel enthused about anything these days." In the last example, the word "rarely" suggests that there may be times when the client feels more enthused than usual. This can prompt detail-gathering questions that explore what is different about those times and how the client helped to bring them about.

Regardless of how constant the problem seems to the client, there are always fluctuations in its frequency and intensity. This means that exceptions are always happening to one degree or another despite the client's difficulty in noticing them. As de Shazer (1991) observed, "times when the complaint is absent are dismissed as trivial by the client or even remain completely unseen, hidden from the client's view" (p. 58)—which is why SFT therapists ask specific questions to elicit exceptions. One of the simplest ways to do this is to ask about small pieces of the client's miracle (or tomorrow) day that have already happened ("What small parts of your miracle day have you noticed lately?").

Here are a few more exception-finding questions and strategies that can be used during or between sessions:

- When is the problem absent or less noticeable?
- When are things are little better between you and your partner?
- Between now and our next meeting, pay attention to anything about your life that you want to continue happening.

Therapists can also discover exceptions by asking about *pretreatment (or presession) changes*, referring to positive changes in the problem situation that occur between the client's decision to seek help and the first therapy session. In an early study by the Milwaukee group, 66% of the 30 clients surveyed said they had noticed pretreatment changes (Weiner-Davis et al., 1987). Although the percentage has been relatively lower in other studies (Ness & Murphy, 2001), pretreatment changes represent useful exceptions that can be elicited in the first session ("Has anything changed for the better, even just a little, since we scheduled this meeting?").

Scaling questions serve many purposes in SFT, one of which is to elicit exceptions. For example, therapists can use the "miracle scale" (de Shazer et al., 2021) to discover exceptions following the client's miracle description. Here is a quick illustration involving Fan, a 55-year-old Chinese client who was struggling with depression and wanted "to feel more energetic and normal like I used to." The dialogue picks up right after Fan had described her postmiracle day.

Therapist: On a scale from 0 to 10, 10 being the day after the miracle you just described and 0 being the exact opposite, where would you put yourself now?

Fan: Uh, 2.5.

Practitioners who are new to SFT may be tempted to ask what a 3 or higher number would look like. However, at this point in the conversation, it is usually more effective—and more likely to elicit exceptions—to ask clients why their rating was not lower and invite them to identify differences between their number and a lower number. Therapists can also ask if the rating has ever been lower and, if so, explore positive differences that explain the client's higher current rating.

Therapist: What is happening differently now that puts you at a 2.5 rather than a 1 or 0?

Fan: I don't know.

Therapist: [pausing to give Fan time to think because this is not the type of question that most clients have considered] It's a tough question. Take your time.

Fan: Well, I'm not missing as much work as I missed last year.

Therapist: Interesting. What else is different now compared to 0? [This was the first of several "What else?" questions aimed at eliciting additional differences, exceptions, and other resources that accounted for Fan's rating of 2.5 rather than a lower number.]

Fan was able to describe a few more exceptions, such as getting along better with a friend, going out for drinks recently with coworkers, and getting a little more sleep during the past week.

Once an exception is identified, therapists explore specifics such as *who* did *what* to make it happen, *when* and *where* it occurred, and other exception-related details. Here are a few detail-gathering questions the therapist asked Fan about the time she joined her coworkers for drinks: "What was different about that time?" "How did you find the energy to do that?" "What does that say about you?" "What will it take to make it happen again?"

In addition to asking these questions, it is useful to find out if the client views an exception as deliberate or random (De Jong & Berg, 2013). If clients are able to link the exception to something they did differently to make it happen, then it is considered a *deliberate exception*. If they are not able to do so, it is called a *random exception*. Random exceptions are often expressed in client responses such as "It just happened," "I don't know what I did differently," and similar statements. The distinction between deliberate and random exceptions is useful to consider when formulating end-of session summaries—which often include invitations to notice and/or expand on exceptions going forward. For example, clients who describe deliberate exceptions might be asked to reflect on what it would take to make them happen more often or in other settings. Clients who report random exceptions may be invited to pay particular attention to their role in making exceptions happen during the coming week.

There are times when clients spontaneously refer to exceptions with no explicit prompting from the therapist, as Rosa does in the following excerpt from the first session.

Therapist: I really appreciate you answering all these questions about what you would be noticing after the miracle [referring to the postmiracle day Rosa had described earlier in the session]. What was it like for you to talk about that?

Rosa: It was good. I think it helped. I mean, I can picture it in my mind. I'm picturing events and times when it has happened.

Rosa's experience of "picturing events and times when it has happened" is not uncommon for clients who are able to describe their preferred futures in sufficient detail. This may be because we tend to visualize what we think about and talk about. Describing hoped-for events and experiences invites clients to picture and "virtually" experience them—which makes it easier for them to recall recent exceptions. Even so, most clients will require more questions and assistance than Rosa did in making the shift from describing their preferred future to remembering recent instances of it. Next, the therapist follows Rosa's lead by exploring the "events and times" she referred to in her previous statement.

Therapist: Tell me about some of those events and times when it has happened? [using Rosa's exact wording]

Rosa: There are times when Mia listens and minds better, and it's easier interacting with her. She's very task oriented when you give her jobs. She loves to help. She craves attention, so when you do give her positive attention, she responds well. If I've got a craft activity planned or I'm baking something she can help with, or playing a game with her, she can be a model child. When we do things like that, it's definitely better. But it's just not always possible to give her the level of attention she craves. That's when she'll find other ways to get attention, and that's when the trouble starts.

Therapist: It's interesting how she responds so well to the positive attention you give her. Like a model child, as you said. That's a high compliment coming from a parent.

Rosa: (*smiles*) Yeah, she's good during those times. She's definitely capable of it.

Therapist: It sounds like you're both capable of making that happen.

Rosa: It's just getting her to be more like that when she's not getting the attention.

Therapist: Yes. So, these events and times are happening, just maybe not as often, or, uh, in as many situations, as you would like?

Rosa: Yes.

Therapist: I'm curious what else you do, or other people do, or anything else that helps make these events and times happen more.

Rosa: Hmm. Let's see. (*pauses*) I mean, we saw that her behavior improved when she started back at school after she was home for a while because of COVID. You know, at the end of the online instruction period [referring to the 3-month period of time when Mia received online instruction at home during the pandemic]. She likes school, so it was good for her to go back. Even though we were a little reluctant to send her back, it's been good for her.

Therapist: Okay. What else seems to help?

Rosa: Getting to bed at a decent time definitely helps me wake up quicker and feel better, you know, more energy, less irritable. I'm more patient with Mia and everybody else. The same for Sal. Sometimes we both stay up too late, and we end up regretting it in the morning. Maybe we'll be able to do that at some point, but not for a while. (*laughs*) There's just a lot going on in the morning.

Therapist: I can't imagine trying to do all that. You only have two hands, right?

Rosa: I can use more, especially in the morning.

Therapist: I'll bet. What else seems to help things go a little better?

Rosa: You mean in the morning?

Therapist: Anytime.

Rosa: Sometimes Sal will play a game, like a card game, with Mia when he gets home from work. I bought them a new card game and Mia loves it. That's what they've been playing in the afternoons. So, something little like that really helps. She looks forward to it, and she'll sit there and play as long as he's willing to. It's great for them, and it gives me time to do other things.

Therapist: Things such as . . .?

Rosa: Relax for a few minutes, do something with the other kids, get dinner started. So, just something little, like playing cards for a few minutes. When we insert them into our day, they seem to make a difference.

Therapist: That's great.

Rosa: That card game was worth every penny. (*laughs*)

Therapist: Sounds like it. It seems like you're already doing some things to be more like you want to be at home. You know, more chill and patient with Mia and others.

Rosa: I guess so.

Since Rosa was able to identify a few deliberate exceptions by describing what she and others had done to bring them about, the therapist's end-of-session summary invited her to continue noticing and building on exceptions and anything else that helped her become a "more chill and patient" person and parent.

Conversations about exceptions often reveal useful inner and outer client resources. For Rosa, these resources included her ability to recognize Mia's strengths ("she can be a model child"); Sal's help and their teamwork during mornings and other times; her solution ideas (getting to bed earlier, having Mia help in the kitchen); sense of humor ("That card game was worth every penny"); and resilience in the face of her parenting challenges, full-time job, and other responsibilities. These resources can be further explored and enlisted in support of Rosa's goal of becoming more patient.

As seen with Rosa, the cultural, social, and personal resources that clients bring to therapy are as unique and varied as clients themselves—and they are there for the asking. With that point in mind, the following client strengths and resources are often available: *resilience and coping abilities* (ability to persevere, cope, and keep going in the face of current and previous struggles); *personal attributes* (caring, courage, kindness, empathy, honesty, humor, and other traits that may enhance the client's achievement of desired outcomes); *prior solutions and solution attempts* (wisdom gained from previous solutions and from current attempts to address the problem); *personal values and worldviews* (cherished values, beliefs, and world views); *solution ideas and theories* (the client's ideas and theories about how change happens for them and how they could improve their situation); *creativity and ingenuity* (the client's creativity and ingenuity in considering different ways to achieve desired outcomes); *personal heroes and influential people* (personal heroes and other respected/ influential people in the client's life—siblings, parents, grandparents, other relatives; friends; authors, celebrities, musicians, athletes, or others whom the client looks up to and respects); *special interests, hobbies, and talents* (cooking, dancing, sports, music, being a good listener or friend to others, and anything else the client is good at, interested in, and enjoys doing); and *social and community supports* (individuals, groups, organizations, or institutions that are important to the client and may assist them in achieving desired outcomes).

In addition to discovering these resources while exploring exceptions, therapists can seek them out during casual opening interactions at the start of therapy ("What do you enjoy doing?" "How did you get good at that?") and other times ("How do keep going with all you've been through?"). Once a useful resource is discovered, therapists can explore how the client might apply it toward desired outcomes just as they would do with an exception. For example, when Rosa was asked how she managed to keep going in the face of her struggles, she discussed the value of family and parenting that was instilled in her by her mother and Latinx culture, adding that this value had helped her handle challenges in her life. She also commented that teaching children to respect adults—another cultural/familial strength and value she brought to therapy—had motivated her to become "the best possible parent" she could be for her children.

Task 3: Exploring Progress

The main purpose of exploring client progress in SFT is to facilitate change-focused conversations related to the client's goal or desired outcome. For example, obtaining the client's 0–10 rating of where they are in relation to their preferred future gives therapists several solution-building options ("Why isn't it lower?" "How did you move up a whole point from last time?" "How have you kept things from getting worse?"). In SFT, exploring progress is broadly defined as measuring and responding to client progress in ways that facilitate change-focused conversations and desired outcomes. The definition includes the following activities: measuring progress; responding to client reports of improvements, no change, or declines; asking about next signs and next steps; and ending therapy.

Measuring Progress

The main means by which SFT practitioners measure client progress and initiate progress-related discussions are by using formal scales (ORS) or informal scaling questions ("On a scale of 0–10 . . ."). For example, progress scales are used to find out where the client is relative to their preferred future, where they would need to be to consider therapy no longer necessary, and how they would know they've moved up during the coming week, to name just a few uses of scales. Although therapists may use other methods (e.g., client checklists, surveys, inventories), scaling remains the most common way of exploring client progress in SFT.

Responding to Client Reports of Improvements, No Change, and Declines

Regardless of whether clients report improvements, no change, or declines, therapists respond by acknowledging their experience and inviting them to describe aspects of their lives that support desired outcomes.

When Clients Report Improvements. The following strategies are useful when clients report improvements from one session to the next:

- *Ask strategy and identity questions.*
  - Strategy questions: What did you do differently to move up a whole point? How did you get yourself to do that? How do you keep going?
  - Identity questions: Where did you find the courage to do that? What do these changes say about you? What have you learned about yourself?
- *Explore social aspects and consequences of improvements*: Who else noticed? How did they react? What was that like for you? How are things different now with your partner?
- *Recruit social support*: Who else might help you maintain these changes? How could you go about getting their help?
- *Request the client's advice*: What tips would you offer to others who want to make similar changes? What would you say to other couples struggling with these challenges?

Although not a standard part of SFT, I occasionally write between-session letters to acknowledge and amplify client improvements. With the client's permission, I have texted and emailed short letters as well as sending them through regular mail. Here is a letter the therapist sent to Rosa between the first and second session:

> Dear Rosa,
>
> I know it's been a tough year for you in many ways, yet you have somehow managed to keep going and doing what you've needed to do for your family, job, and other parts of your life. I appreciated your patience and cooperation in answering my questions about what you wanted from our meetings. Your detailed miracle description helped me better understand you and your hopes for the future. I invite you to continue noticing and perhaps even making a list of any small pieces of the miracle that are already happening, along with anything you do to help make them happen. I look forward to our next meeting.

The following conversation occurred during the early moments of the second and final session with Rosa.

Therapist: Where would you put yourself on the 0-to-10 scale from last time, where 10 means you're right where you want to be as a parent, and 0 is the exact opposite of that?

Rosa: Uh, I'd say about 7.

Therapist: That's 4 points higher than last time. How did you make that happen? [strategy question]

Rosa described several positive changes that were helping her become the person and parent she wanted to be. These changes included setting out her children's clothes the night before school, going to bed a little earlier, setting her alarm to wake up 20 or 30 minutes before waking the kids, and occasionally initiating a game or craft with Mia in the evening. Of all these changes, waking up before the kids on school days made the biggest difference according to Rosa. The therapist listened as she described these and other improvements, occasionally asking a question to clarify Rosa's contributions and other progress-related details.

Therapist: How did you get yourself to wake up before the kids?

Rosa: It's not easy. (*laughs*) I told my husband we needed to go to bed earlier to have a fighting chance in the mornings. We don't always do it, but we're getting better. And I'm in a better mood.

Therapist: How so?

Rosa: Just being able to sit and breathe a little in the morning, have a cup of coffee in peace before the chaos starts. It puts me in a more positive mindset.

A few minutes later:

Therapist: You've done a lot to help yourself, Rosa. What have these changes taught you about yourself? [identity question]

Rosa: That I can be more chill with Mia, my kids, my husband.

Therapist: Is that a new, uh, realization, or something you've known all along?

Rosa: Hmm. I think I knew it, because I've felt it before, even when Mia was flipping out about something. But those moments were far and few between. (*laughs*)

Therapist: And they're happening more now?

Rosa: Yes. I still have a way to go, but it's better than it was a few weeks ago. For me, it's a matter of being more intentional about things. You know, taking a breath to think, "How do I want to respond to this?" before jumping in and just reacting.

When Clients Report No Change or Declines. Clients tend to report between-session improvements more often than not, but there are certainly times when they don't. Even though exceptions have most likely occurred between sessions, it is hard for clients to notice them in the midst of their difficulties. The following ideas are useful to consider when responding to clients who report that things have stayed the same or become worse.

Although therapists naturally want clients to improve and may be disheartened when they don't, it is important to keep these feelings in check when responding to clients in these situations. SFT practitioners do this by adopting a both/and position that acknowledges the client's problems *and* possibilities. Students or practitioners new to SFT are prone to prematurely asking about exceptions before properly acknowledging the client's disappointment and frustration or to trying to convince clients that progress *must* have occurred ("Surely something has been better since our last session, right?"). These responses tend to impede the alliance and stifle progress because the client may feel unheard and perceive the therapist as minimizing the seriousness of the situation. Acknowledging clients' frustrations strengthens the alliance and paves the way for exploring resilience and other resources that support desired outcomes.

Coping questions invite clients to reflect on personal attributes and actions that have helped them persist in the face of difficulties and keep things from getting worse. Examples include "How do you keep going?"

"With everything you've been through, how have you held things together and stayed at it for so long?" and "How have you stopped things from getting worse?" These questions validate clients' struggles and invite them to describe actions, qualities, and other resources that enable them to cope with difficulties and keep going.

When Therapy Stops Working. The following options are useful to consider when clients do not report any improvements for two or more consecutive sessions (Murphy, 2023).

- **Ask the client.** Request the client's feedback on getting unstuck and turning things around ("What can I do differently, or we do differently, to make this more useful for you?"). Therapists who use the SRS can discuss the client's ratings for similar troubleshooting purposes.
- **Examine the desired outcome.** *Is there a clearly stated, agreed-upon goal or desired outcome?* If not, it needs to be developed; If so, therapists can explore its achievability and importance. *Achievability*: "On a scale of 0 to 10, with 10 meaning you are very confident that you can achieve (desired outcome) and 0 being the opposite, where would you rate it?" If the rating is low, invite the client to revise the outcome to make it more attainable. If the rating is midrange or high, explore what is contributing to the client's confidence and what next signs or next steps might inspire even more confidence in achieving the outcome. *Importance*: "On a 0–10 scale, where 10 means [desired outcome] is extremely important to you and 0 is the exact opposite, where would you rate it?" If low, renegotiate an outcome that is more important to the client. If high, explore how willing the client is to take steps toward achieving the outcome: "On a 0–10 scale, where 10 means 'I'll do anything' to reach [desired outcome] and 0 means the opposite, . . .?" *Has the outcome changed?* Sometimes the client's desired outcome has changed unbeknownst to the therapist. This can result in working at cross-purposes with one another, which is why it is important to check in with the client at the start of second and later sessions to see if the desired outcome has changed.
- **Change things up.** Consider changing session schedules, times, formats, and participants. Examples include switching from weekly to biweekly

meetings, from evening to morning sessions, from sitting during the entire meeting to occasionally standing or walking, and from meeting the client individually to including others in the session.

- **Consult with colleagues.** Consult with colleagues for ideas on getting unstuck. With the client's consent, consider inviting a colleague to serve as a cotherapist or to observe a live or taped session and offer feedback. If these options are not feasible, conduct a virtual or imaginary consultation with a respected mentor to stimulate new ideas and options.
- **Change the approach.** No single therapy approach works for every client. If nothing changes after trying the above options, then try a different approach that might fit better for the client. For therapists who use the SRS, the client's feedback and comments related to the "Approach or Method" item may be helpful in choosing a different approach.
- **Change therapists.** Just as any single approach is not effective for all clients, the best of therapists will not be effective with every client. If the client shows no progress after these strategies have been implemented, recommend a different therapist. If that is not possible, take a break from the schedule to reexamine the situation and resume therapy with a renewed sense of hope.

Asking About Next Signs and Next Steps

Solution-focused therapists periodically ask about *next signs* of further progress ("What will be the first small signs of progress?") and *next steps* in that direction ("What small step might help make that happen?"). These questions are often incorporated into end-of-session summaries or messages for clients. Although both questions are used in SFT, there is a distinction to consider when choosing which one to ask. Questions about next signs invite clients to reflect, which is a relatively benign activity that clients generally accept. Questions about next steps require clients to describe specific strategies or actions they could take to move forward. This may fit well for clients who want to leave the session with an action plan, but not for those who, for whatever reason, are not ready to take specific steps or actions.

Ending Therapy

Measuring and exploring client progress figure prominently in decisions about ending therapy. SFT practitioners invite clients to *begin with the end in mind* by selecting a "good enough" point on the scale to end therapy. When clients reach or exceed this point, therapists initiate a discussion about terminating services. This is a collaborative decision, and clients are given an open invitation to contact the practitioner and resume therapy as needed in the future.

In the final session with Rosa, she put herself at 7 on the 0–10 miracle/ preferred future scale and described several recent improvements that accounted for the high number. Rosa's rating, which was 4 points higher than it was at the start of therapy, matched the "good enough" number she wanted to be at to end therapy. The following conversation occurred toward the end of the session.

Therapist: After hearing about all these changes and the effects they've had for you and Mia and the whole family, I can understand why your rating climbed to a 7.

Rosa: I just hope I can keep it up.

Therapist: Yeah. What would help you keep it up in the future? [using Rosa's words to explore her ideas for maintaining progress]

Rosa: Just keep doing what I'm doing now, I guess.

Therapist: Okay.

Rosa: But I'm a little worried about that.

Therapist: Worried about . . .?

Rosa: You know, just continuing to do these things that are working now, like getting to bed on time, laying out clothes, that's a tough one, and the other stuff I mentioned. I get pretty wound up when I have a lot going on, and I don't want to backslide into old habits.

Therapist: That makes sense.

The next few minutes were spent discussing ideas for maintaining progress and handling inevitable slips and setbacks along the way. This discussion seemed to bolster Rosa's faith in her ability to sustain progress, which was verified by her confidence rating below.

Therapist: On a scale of 0 to 10, where 10 means you're fully confident in continuing the changes you've made, and 0 means the opposite, where would you put yourself now?

Rosa: I'd say, uh, around 6.5 or 7. I mean, I know I won't remember to do certain things just because life happens, and we forget to use the skills we have. Just because Mia's doing better now doesn't mean something won't come up next week with her or one of the other kids. But I'd like to think I'll recognize when I start stressing out and do something about it. I'd be foolish not to.

Therapist: Not to . . . ?

Rosa: Keep doing this stuff. I mean, it's helping me, Mia, all of us. So, I want to keep it up.

Therapist: Okay. And, like you said, there are no guarantees that things won't be more challenging next week or whenever. But at least you have some ideas for handling those times when they happen.

Rosa: I'm sure they'll happen. I just don't want things to go back to where they were last month.

The above conversation laid the groundwork for exploring the possibility of ending therapy, which is where the following dialogue picks just a few minutes before the session ended.

Therapist: In our first meeting, I asked what number on the scale would be good enough for you to consider ending therapy. Do you happen to remember what you said?

Rosa: 7 or 8, I think.

Therapist: Yes, you said "between a 7 or 8." So, I'm wondering what you would think about taking a break from meeting for now, knowing we can resume things anytime you want to in the future.

Rosa: That's funny. I was thinking of that on the way here. The thing is, I know what I need to do. Maybe I've always known. It's just a matter of doing it, which is easier said than done.

Therapist: Yes, it is.

Therapy was discontinued that day and Rosa has not contacted the therapist to resume it.

As illustrated with Rosa, SFT conversations about ending therapy frequently involve comparing the client's initial rating on the 0–10 miracle/preferred future scale with their current and "good enough" ratings, highlighting the client's successes and contributions to progress, obtaining the client's input on ending services, and exploring what it will take to sustain progress. Giving the client a central voice in ending therapy is based on a simple idea: If the therapist believes the client when they say they need therapy, then they should believe them when they say they no longer need it.

For clients who are concerned about losing the gains they've made, therapists validate their concerns and collaborate on plans for preventing slips and responding effectively should they occur. One advantage of SFT when it comes to ending services is that therapists position themselves and their services as peripheral versus central parts of the client's life. Attributing progress to the client's efforts and contributions enhances their ownership and maintenance of therapy gains. The decentralized role of solution-focused therapists also makes it less likely that clients will become overly dependent on the therapist or therapy.

CORE TECHNIQUES

SFT techniques fall into three interrelated categories: *asking* useful questions, *listening* closely to clients' responses, and *amplifying* aspects of their responses and lives that support desired outcomes. When being purely solution-focused, there is rarely anything the therapist does outside of these three activities.

Listening

Listening is important in all therapy approaches. However, *what* the therapist listens for and responds to is different for different approaches. As Lipchik (2002) noted, solution-focused therapists listen for signs of exceptions, resilience, hope, competency, progress, and anything else that supports desired outcomes: "We do not ignore anything we hear, but at the same time, we only respond to what is potentially useful for the client" (p. 44). De Jong and Berg (2013) use the phrase "listen, select, and build" to describe SFT's coconstructive process of listening for hints of possibility and asking follow-up questions to explore and amplify pieces of clients' responses and lives that support their therapy goals.

Asking

Questions are the primary means by which therapists initiate conversations in SFT. Most of the questions therapists ask are constructed from the client's previous answer and often incorporate the client's key words and phrases. This section describes several frequently used questions in SFT.

Difference Questions

Difference questions seek to elicit and explore meaningful differences related to the client's desired outcome. Examples include differences between the client's present situation and preferred future ("If a miracle occurred tonight, what would be different about tomorrow?"), exceptions and other times ("What was different about the time you were calmer than usual?"), and lower and higher scale ratings ("What's different now that you're at a 4 compared with last time when you were at a 2.5?").

Instead Questions

Clients who are asked what they want from therapy frequently describe what they do *not* want, or want less of, in their lives ("I want to be less depressed"; "We want to stop arguing so much"). When this occurs, solution-focused therapists ask *instead questions* to encourage clients to describe what they want instead ("What would you rather be feeling/doing instead?").

Due to the way language works, it is difficult to talk about feeling "less depressed" without thinking about depression or picturing being depressed. This is one reason solution-focused therapists invite people to describe what they want *more of* versus less of. Another reason is because it is much harder to observe and describe something that is not there (e.g., less depression or absence of depression) compared with something that is, such as cooking a meal or being on time for work. Clients tend to become more energized when working *toward* a positively stated outcome than "away from" a negatively stated one. "Instead questions" invite clients to describe what they want in positive, observable terms.

Relationship Questions

Clients exist in social systems that include key people, relationships, and interactions. In addition to involving significant others in therapy sessions, we can ask *relationship questions* that invite clients to consider their current situation, preferred future, and progress toward that future from the perspective of others:

- Who will be the first ones to notice you being more patient? How will they respond? What will that be like for you?
- Who else might help you sustain these changes? How can you get their help?
- How will your friends know you're more patient?

Strategy and Identity Questions

As seen with Rosa, strategy questions invite clients to describe actions and efforts that contribute to their progress and exceptions ("How did you make that happen? What have you done differently to move 4 points higher?"). Identity questions invite clients to describe personal attributes and meanings associated with exceptions or progress ("What did you draw on to make it happen? What does that say about you?"). These questions credit clients for positive changes and make it less likely that they will attribute the changes to luck, fate, or other factors unrelated to their own actions and attributes.

Coping Questions

Coping questions are used throughout SFT and play a key role when clients report a decline or lack of change from one session to the next ("With all you've been through, how do you manage to keep going?" "Where do you find the strength to stay at it through all these challenges?"). As seen in these examples, coping questions often acknowledge clients' difficulties ("With all you've been through, . . .") and invite them to describe how they are coping and managing (". . . how do you manage to keep going?").

Scaling Questions

Scaling questions are used in every phase of SFT from setting a direction ("What would be a 'good enough' number on the 0–10 scale for you to end therapy?") through exploring progress ("How did you get from 5 to 7?"). As seen in the client examples, defining 0 in vague terms ("the opposite of being patient") rather than specific terms ("being short with your kids") makes it more likely to get a response above 0—which enables therapists to explore differences between 0 and the client's higher rating.

Appendix A includes these and other questions that solution-focused therapists use in setting a direction, building on exceptions and other resources, and exploring progress.

Amplifying

Amplifying, which often takes the form of questions, is defined as expanding something in size or importance by the use of detail, illustration, or closer analysis (Merriam-Webster, n.d.). This definition also captures the overall nature of SFT, which can be viewed as the process of amplifying what clients want from therapy and what they already have toward achieving it.

Amplifying often involves exploring details about clients' hopes and goals, exceptions and resources, and progress toward desired outcomes. One of the most common ways to do this is to ask, "What else?"—which may be the most frequently asked question in SFT. Other forms of amplifying include *making lists* ("Let's make a list of 10 or more people who want the best for you and might be willing to help you become more patient"); *acknowledging* and *validating* ("No wonder you feel so bad with everything you've been through"); *echoing* the client's words ("What else has been helping you become 'more chill and patient' at home?"); *complimenting* ("Mia is lucky to have you in her corner"); and *summarizing* clients' hopes, resources, and progress in end-of session summaries and occasionally during the session.

SESSION STRUCTURE

The following components and sequences of first and later sessions in SFT are general guidelines that are flexibly applied to fit the client and situation.

First Session

1. **Opening.** In addition to completing introductions and paperwork requirements, therapists can ask about nonproblem topics including the client's work, hobbies, and special interests ("What do you like doing in your spare time?" "How did you get good at that?"). Although these conversations are optional in SFT, they may help clients ease into the session by discussing topics that are familiar and interesting to them. In addition to revealing resources that may come in handy later, these conversations convey the therapist's appreciation of the client as a person apart from the problem.

2. **Setting a direction.** This step typically involves determining what the client wants from therapy (desired outcome), eliciting a detailed description of how their lives would be different if they were to achieve it (preferred future/solution description), and obtaining a 0–10 rating of where they are in relation to their preferred future and where they would need to be in order to end therapy.

3. **Building on exceptions and other resources.** Setting a direction naturally leads to exploring exceptions and other resources that support the client's desired outcome.

4. **Exploring progress.** Although exploring progress plays a larger role in second and later sessions, therapists may ask a few progress-related questions in the first session to see where clients put themselves on the miracle/preferred future scale and to explore pretreatment changes ("Has anything improved since you scheduled this meeting?") and "next signs" of future progress ("How will you know you've moved up on the scale?").

5. **Closing.** Some solution-focused therapists take a short break toward the end of each session to gather their thoughts and prepare a summary statement or message for clients (De Jong & Berg, 2013). Regardless of whether one takes a break or not, closing summaries usually include acknowledgement and appreciation of the client's cooperation, struggles, perseverance, hopes, motivations, exceptions, and other aspects of their lives that support desired outcomes. Therapists might also suggest between-session tasks or experiments for clients to consider, such as being on the lookout for exceptions, noticing any signs of progress, taking small steps toward desired outcomes, and noticing anything else in their lives that support desired outcomes. I end most sessions by asking clients if I missed any important questions or topics, if or when they want to meet again, and if they could help me out by completing the SRS.

Later Sessions

Therapists usually begin second and later sessions by asking, "What's better?" or by using formal or informal 0–10 scales (ORS or "Where are you on the 0–10 miracle scale?"). When clients report gains, therapists ask how they made it happen, who noticed, and what else has been different since their recent progress. When things have declined or stayed the same, therapists ask clients how they've managed to keep going and what might help turn things around. Barring a change in the client's desired outcome, the session would then proceed through modified versions of Steps 3 through 5 above.

CLIENT ILLUSTRATION: JALEN

Jalen, a 27-year-old African American client, entered therapy at the suggestion of a social worker (Rita) from a local homeless shelter where he had previously lived. He left the shelter and rented a small apartment in the same town, where he had been living for 2 months before starting therapy. Rita told me Jalen experienced a traumatic childhood and adolescence characterized by physical abuse from his father, intermittent periods of homelessness, and several interruptions in his formal education. She added that his "social anxiety was flaring up again" and that he spent most of his time inside the apartment.

The therapist met with Jalen four times over a period of 8 weeks. The dialogues and commentaries in this illustration focus primarily on the first session because it is the most challenging phase of SFT, particularly for students and practitioners who are new to the approach.

Session One

Jalen completed the ORS and other required forms a few minutes before the first session. The following conversation occurred after introductions and the therapist's orienting comments about the purpose and process of therapy (". . . helping you get what you want from this, which means I'll need to ask you some questions").

Therapist: It would help me to get to know you a little better by learning what you enjoy doing.

Jalen: Hmm. (*pauses for several seconds*)

Therapist: Just anything you like doing for fun or are good at.

Jalen: I like video games, especially the ones where you have to travel someplace and bad guys are trying to stop you.

Therapist: Are you pretty good at those games?

Jalen: People tell me I am.

Therapist: How did you get good at it?

Jalen explained how he got progressively better at two video games. He also said he was a "great babysitter" for his nieces and nephew, who often request having him instead of other babysitters.

Therapist: What is it about you that makes you a great babysitter? [This "identity question" invites Jalen to describe personal attributes, actions, or other resources that enhance his effectiveness as a babysitter—and might help him achieve desired outcomes.]

Jalen said he was a "cool babysitter" because he joked around with the kids and let them have fun. He made the following comment just as the therapist was about ask what he wanted from therapy.

Jalen: A few years ago, someone asked me where I saw myself in 10 years. I said, "I don't."

(*The therapist and Jalen were silent for several seconds.*)

Jalen: I wasn't even supposed to make it to 25.

Therapist: (*pauses*) And yet you did.

Jalen: I did. I wasn't sure I would. I've been through some tough times.

Jalen went on to describe previous challenges that included physical abuse from his father, seeking shelter on his own as an adolescent, missing meals because there was no food in the house, and recent periods of home-lessness. After acknowledging these challenges, the therapist asked Jalen how he managed to "make it to 25" with all he had been through.

Jalen: I don't know, I just did it.

Therapist: You just did it. What helped you do it?

Jalen: I don't know. What choice did I have? Either sleep on the park bench or freeze to death sleeping on the ground. You got to do what you got to do. That's just the way it is.

Therapist: Well, not everyone who faces those things gets through them like you have.

Jalen: I just did what I had to do. But I think it affected me, you know? Like the problems I'm having now.

Therapist: Yes. Well, as I said earlier, I want this meeting to be useful for you. So, if it is, what would be noticing to tell you it was useful?

Jalen: I think having someone to talk to, someone who will listen, will help. [As seen earlier with Rosa and now Jalen, clients may respond to desired outcome questions by referring to in-session processes or activities, such as "talking things out" or "getting things off my chest." When this occurs, solution-focused therapists incorporate clients' words into follow-up questions designed to elicit a hoped-for outcome "outside" of the therapy session—because that is where they live their lives.]

Therapist: Let's say we talked things out here and it helped. What would you be doing differently, or feeling differently, or anything else, when you leave here, that would tell you or others that it was a good idea to meet with me today?

Jalen: (*pauses*) I'd be getting out into it.

Therapist: Getting out into it.

Jalen: You know, getting out of the house and seeing more people. Being more social, I guess.

Therapist: Being more social. Okay. So, which of these marks will go up most when you become more social? (*pointing to Jalen's completed ORS*)

Jalen: Um, these two [pointing to the Interpersonally (family, intimate relationships) and Socially (work, school, peers) items which he rated as 5.3 and 3.6, respectively. Both items were relatively lower than his Individually (personal well-being) rating of 6.5 and Overall rating of 6.2. His total score on the ORS was 21.6].

Therapist: Which one is most important to you?

Jalen: This one. (*pointing to his mark of 3.6 on the Socially item*)

Therapist: Okay. And what spot or number on this line would you need to be at to feel like you got what you wanted from this and no longer needed to meet with me?

Jalen: That's a tough one. (*pauses for several seconds*) Up around here somewhere, maybe around 8.

Therapist: Thank you. That's helpful. I have another hard question that will take some imagination. Imagine that you wake up tomorrow and this line is way up here (*pointing toward the highest spot on the Socially line of Jalen's ORS form*) and that you're getting out into it and being social exactly the way you want to. Okay?

Jalen: (*nods "yes"*)

Therapist: What is the very first thing you would notice tomorrow morning to tell you things are different and better?

Jalen: I'd wake up. Does that count?

Therapist: Yes, that counts. What else would you notice?

For the next several minutes, the therapist and Jalen struggled to construct a more detailed description of what it would look if he was being more social. At one point, Jalen apologized because he was not answering the questions right. The therapist reassured him that he was doing fine and that many people struggle with these questions because they are hard to answer. Jalen seemed to relax a bit, and the therapist took a different approach to eliciting his preferred future as seen below.

Therapist: Do you like movies?

Jalen: I love movies.

Therapist: Me, too. If you're willing to try something a little strange, I wonder if you can imagine that you're sitting in a movie theatre, okay? (*Jalen nods "yes."*) You've got a great seat and the movie is about to start. You can even close your eyes if you want to, but you don't have to. (*Jalen closes his eyes.*) The strange thing is that this movie is about your life 3 months from now—3 months into the future—when you're more social and your life is much closer to the way you want it to be. Tell me about one or more of the scenes from this movie.

Jalen described several scenes that included different people, settings, and situations. The therapist made a list of key scenes and details for future reference. As the session was about to end, the therapist offered the following message:

Therapist: With everything you've been through, it's inspiring that you've managed to keep going and stay at it. Your decision to talk with me today is another example of your effort to make things better. I appreciate your patience in answering all my questions and teaching me more about your hope of being more social—and about what it would look like when you do. So, between now and next time we meet, maybe you could be on the lookout for small parts of those movie scenes that are happening in your life, even just a tiny bit. Does that make sense? (*Jalen nods "yes."*) Okay. I just need your help on another short form that tells me how this meeting went for you [referring to the SRS]. Can you help me with that?

Jalen's SRS ratings were as follows: (a) Relationship (feeling heard and respected)—9.7, Goals and Topics (importance of topics discussed)—9.5, Approach or Method (goodness of fit between therapist's approach and client)—9.6, Overall (overall effectiveness of session)—9.3, and Total score—38.1. Although these ratings suggest a sufficiently strong client–therapist alliance, the therapist asked if there was anything else he or they could do differently next time to make the session more useful. Jalen said "no" and added: "It's nice to be asked your opinion of things. Nobody asks me what I think about things, they usually just tell me what I should be doing or not doing. I've heard that all my life."

Jalen's comments reinforce the solution-focused practice of asking versus telling or assuming. Asking for clients' feedback and adjusting services in accordance with their feedback is one of several ways solution-focused therapists put cultural humility and cultural responsiveness into action. Instead of telling clients what to do or not do based on the therapist's assessment or therapy model, solution-focused therapists ask questions that encourage clients to develop their own solutions. All clients appreciate being asked for their opinions and perceptions, especially if they are from underrepresented groups as Jalen was.

The therapist thanked Jalen for his feedback and asked if or when he wanted to meet again (another difference between SFT and other approaches in which the between-session interval is determined primarily by the therapist). They decided to meet in 2 weeks.

Session Two

Jalen's ratings on the ORS—which he completed in the waiting room prior to the session—declined slightly from his original ratings as follows: Individually (5.7, a .8 decline), Interpersonally (4.7, a .6 decline), Socially (3.2, a .4 decline), Overall (5.3, a .9 decline), and Total score (18.9, a 2.7 decline).

Therapist: Before talking about this [pointing to Jalen's completed ORS], I'm wondering what's been better since we met last time?

Jalen: Uh, not much. It's been a bad week.

Therapist: A bad week.

Jalen: Yeah, I had a big argument with my sister. It's been brewing for a while, and it finally happened this week. She blames me for problems in her life that I don't have anything to do with. I finally got fed up and told her she needed to get herself together and stop blaming me.

Therapist: How has that affected your ratings in these areas (*pointing to Jalen's completed ORS*)?

Jalen said his problems with his sister explained his lower ORS ratings and "pretty much ruined the week." Next, the therapist asks Jalen how he kept things from getting worse.

Therapist: It sounds like a really tough week, Jalen. Things were hard enough for you before this argument with your sister, which makes me wonder how you've stopped these numbers from going even lower.

Jalen: I don't know. It doesn't seem like I'm doing anything right these days.

Therapist: Okay. Well, thinking back over the past few months or even the past year, was there ever a time when these marks would have been lower?

Jalen: Definitely. A few times in the last year. I mean, I was homeless for almost 6 months and now I have my own apartment.

Therapist: Okay. So, having your own apartment is one reason the numbers are higher now compared to then?

Jalen: (*nods "yes"*)

Therapist: What else explains the higher marks now compared to then?

Without minimizing or invalidating Jalen's current struggles, these coping and exception-finding questions invited him to describe small successes, skills, and other resources that have helped him manage previous difficulties and keep things from getting worse. The remainder of the conversation explored exceptions and other resources that supported his hope of "getting out in it" and becoming more social.

Exceptions to Jalen's self-described "antisocial problem" included two recent trips to the grocery store; a few phone calls with his mother and Rita (the social worker from the homeless shelter); and a grocery store conversation with Claire, a person he knew from the local church he attended while living at the shelter. The therapist asked strategy and identity questions about Jalen's specific contributions to the exceptions ("How did you get yourself to do that?" "What does that say about you?"). Jalen's response to these and other strengths-based questions revealed inner and outer resources that included occasional self-reminders of what he had already overcome to stay alive and have his own apartment, a desire to help others who had experienced homelessness, a "weird" sense of humor, and friends from the church he used to attend.

When Jalen mentioned friends, the therapist invited him to name every person in his life who cared about him and wanted the best for him. Jalen was visibly surprised and pleased when his list exceeded 10, then 15, then 20 before finally stopping at 23 people. At one point toward the end of the list, he said, "I didn't realize there were so many people." When asked about someone on the list who might help him become more social, he mentioned Claire, the person he recently spoke with at the grocery store.

The therapist offered the following summary at the end of the session:

> Although it's been a very tough week, you've once again managed to get through it and keep things from getting worse. You've done a lot to get from where you were last year to where you are now with your own apartment. You've also shown that you're capable of being more social based on the phone calls you've had with Rita and your mother, trips to the grocery store, and your conversation with Claire. It might help to continue noticing these things and other things that help you 'get out in it.' We also talked about all the people in your life, 23 and counting, who care about you and want you to succeed. That's quite a team, Jalen, and it's encouraging to hear that you have all those people in your corner and on your side. You also mentioned the possibility of reaching out to Claire for some help and support. I'll be curious how that goes if you decide to do it.

Jalen rated all four SRS items at 10. The therapist thanked him for his cooperation, asked if he wanted to meet again, and scheduled the next session for 3 weeks from then. The therapist sent Jalen the following letter a few days later to formally acknowledge his resilience, exceptions, and other resources that supported his goal of becoming more social:

> Dear Jalen,
>
> It was good talking with you last week. It is clear that you have done many things to help yourself get through some tough times and to support your hope of being more social. I was also struck by how many people care about you and want the best for you (we listed 23 people). I'll be curious how it goes with Claire if you decide to reach out to her. I invite you to continue noticing any small signs of getting out in it along with anything else that is helping you become more social. You can even make a list of these things for our next meeting if you want to.

Session Three

Jalen's progress ratings on the ORS were markedly higher than his ratings from the previous session as follows: Individually (6.9, a 1.2 increase),

Interpersonally (5.5, a .8 increase), Socially (8.3, a 5.1 increase), Overall (7.0, a 1.7 increase), and Total score (27.7; an 8.8 increase).

Therapist: Wow, Jalen. Your ratings in every area are higher than they were 3 weeks ago, and your total score is over 8 points higher. How would you explain that? [This open-ended question invites a wide range of possible responses.]

Jalen: (*smiles*) A lot of things have been happening, and most of it is good.

Therapist: What's been good lately?

For the next 30 minutes or so, Jalen described several events and activities that accounted for his higher ratings, which included taking Claire up on her invitation to talk by phone (which they did four or five times according to Jalen) and to attend a weekly discussion group involving young adults at the local church (which he did twice). He also called his mother and they had "a decent conversation," and she called him a few days after that. He went to the grocery store several times, including once when he just "felt like getting out" and couldn't think of anywhere else to go. Rita asked if he could periodically help serve evening meals to residents at the shelter—which he did on two occasions since the previous session.

The therapist mostly listened as Jalen talked, occasionally asking a strategy, identity, or relationship question to clarify his contributions to recent exceptions and progress ("How did you do that?" "Where did you find the courage to call Claire/attend the church group/help out at the shelter?" "What does that say about you?" "Who else noticed these differences?"). As Jalen discussed specific differences and improvements, the therapist adhered to the guideline *Never show more enthusiasm about progress than the client does.* Overly enthusiastic therapist responses are uncomfortable for some clients and may unwittingly pressure them into reporting improvements for the therapist's benefit—which is incompatible with SFT's emphasis on the decentralized role of the therapist and the client's ownership of successful outcomes.

A few minutes before the session ended, the therapist broached the topic of ending therapy. This decision was based on Jalen's rating of 8.3 on the ORS Socially item, which is where he wanted to be to end therapy. Jalen acknowledged his progress but was reluctant to discontinue therapy for fear of "relapsing" to where he was a month or so ago. The therapist honored Jalen's preference and they decided to meet in 3 weeks.

The end-of-session summary included the following: acknowledgment of Jalen's resilience and perseverance ("You just keep going and going"); invitation to continue noticing actions, situations, thoughts, feelings, and anything else associated with being social ("I'd suggest continuing to watch for those better times and for what you do to make them happen . . ."); and next signs of further progress (". . . along with paying attention to other small signs or differences that tell you you're on the right track, if that make sense to you"). Jalen's SRS ratings were similar to those of previous sessions, which suggested that he experienced a strong client–therapist alliance and found the session to be useful.

Session Four

Three weeks later, the therapist opened the session by asking, "What's better?" Jalen reported that he had continued many of the changes discussed in the prior session. These changes included attending the young adults group; staying in touch with Claire and a few others from the group; volunteering at the homeless shelter; and leaving the apartment almost every day, once for a job interview at a local restaurant. He added another evening of volunteer work at the shelter and said he enjoyed discussing mutual experiences and challenges with the shelter's residents.

The therapist and Jalen discussed his ORS ratings in light of the above changes and progress. Jalen's ratings, in comparison with his third session ratings, were as follows: Individually (7.2, a .3 increase), Interpersonally (6.1, a .6 increase), Socially (8.6, a .3 increase), Overall (7.5, a .5 increase), and Total score (29.4, a 1.7 increase). Jalen's primary area of concern (Socially) increased by 5 points (from 3.6 to 8.6) since the start of therapy, and he reported progress in every other area of the ORS. The therapist asked strategy, identity, relationship, and other questions to explore and empower Jalen's progress ("How did you get yourself to do that?" "What have you learned about yourself?" "Who else has noticed?" "What advice would you offer someone else who is struggling with becoming more social?").

As the session was about to end, the therapist revisited the possibility of discontinuing therapy because it was the second consecutive session in which Jalen met his "good enough" rating of 8 on the ORS Socially scale.

Therapist: You've done a lot over the past couple of months to become more social, and I wanted to check in with you again to see what you thought about stopping our meetings for the time being, knowing we can pick up again in the future any time you want to.

Jalen: (*pauses for several seconds*) I'll give it a try. I can call you if I start slipping down or anything like that, right?

Therapist: Absolutely.

Jalen never did call back. When the therapist saw Rita several months later, she reported that Jalen was "hanging in there" and had continued to maintain his apartment, volunteer at the shelter, and sustain several other social activities he started during the therapy process.

SUMMARY

Chapter 4 examined the SFT process by describing the role of the therapist, client, and therapeutic relationship, and illustrating SFT in action with a variety of clients and problems. Two extended examples involving clients from underrepresented populations (Rosa and Jalen) demonstrated the implementation of SFT from start to finish across several sessions. As seen with both clients, solution-focused therapists maintain a culturally humble stance by collaborating with clients on the three main tasks of SFT: *setting a direction* for therapy (becoming a more chill and patient parent for Rosa, becoming more social for Jalen), *building on exceptions and other resources* that support clients' desired outcomes (instances of effective parenting and the importance of family for Rosa, trips to the grocery store and a desire to help others for Jalen), and *exploring progress* toward desired outcomes (asking Rosa how she moved from 3 to 7 on the 0–10 scale and asking Jalen how he moved from 21.6 to the 29.4 on the ORS).

The chapter's client examples and transcripts illustrated the three main techniques used by solution-focused therapists: *asking* useful questions, *listening* carefully to clients' responses, and *amplifying* features of their responses and lives that supported their desired outcomes. Chapter 4 also discussed commonly used questions in SFT, such as strategy, identity, difference, and scaling questions, to name a few. The general structure of first and later sessions in SFT was also presented and illustrated through client examples. Chapter 5 examines the evaluation of SFT, a topic that has been integral to the approach's development throughout its history.

5

Evaluation

Solution-focused therapy (SFT) was born out of a discussion of evaluation and evidence-based practice, both of which have been central to
the approach's development, evolution, and credibility. Dissatisfied with
the results of traditional psychotherapy approaches, the Milwaukee group
began to research a more efficient, client-centered approach to therapy.

From the 1980s to the present, SFT developers and researchers have
prioritized client outcomes and real-time client evaluation when measuring the effectiveness of therapy and determining what to keep, dis-
card, and modify in SFT. This inductive, developmental, evidence-based
approach to the construction of solution-focused theory and therapy sets it
apart from other approaches. Unfortunately, the evidence-based origins of
SFT are often overlooked in psychotherapy textbooks and graduate classes
in which SFT is discussed. This chapter describes outcome research on
the effectiveness of SFT, process research on solution-focused practice,

https://doi.org/10.1037/0000370-005
Solution-Focused Therapy, by J. J. Murphy

common factors research as it applies to SFT, transcultural evaluation of SFT, and frequently cited criticisms and potential disadvantages of SFT.

OUTCOME RESEARCH ON THE EFFECTIVENESS OF SFT

Outcome research on the impact of SFT has consistently evolved and expanded since the early days of the Milwaukee group. As a result, the evidence base for SFT has been established across a wide range of clients, concerns, and cultures.

Early Studies

The earliest studies of SFT by the Milwaukee group involved a diverse range of clients and problems that included adults, children, couples, and difficulties ranging from depression and anxiety through domestic violence, relationship problems, substance misuse, school difficulties, and others. These studies were exploratory, qualitative, and practice-based—an approach that was well-suited to the initial stages of therapy development. In one study, de Shazer et al. (1986) reported a 72% success rate for SFT based on a short survey that asked clients if they met their therapy goals. Another study found that 82% of clients surveyed 6 to 18 months after services ended said that therapy was successful (de Shazer, 1985). De Jong and Hopwood (1996) reported on 136 Brief Family Therapy Center clients seen in 1992 and 1993. When asked 7 to 9 months after therapy whether they had met their goals, 45% of clients reported meeting them, 32% reported some progress, and 23% reported no progress.

In addition to researching the overall effectiveness of SFT, the Milwaukee team examined the impact of specific interventions and techniques. In a study of the "formula first session task" (de Shazer, 1985) in which clients are asked to observe specific aspects of their lives they want to continue happening, 50 of 56 new clients (89%) reported that something desirable had happened, with 46 (82%) of them reporting that at least one such event was "new or different" (p. 155). The group also investigated the prevalence of pretreatment (or presession) change, which refers to desired change that occurs between the client's decision to seek formal assistance and the first therapy session. Twenty of 30 new clients (66%) reported pretreatment changes (Weiner-Davis et al., 1987). Although these studies did not use rigorous experimental designs, they provided practice-based evidence grounded in client feedback and self-report—a strategy that remains central to SFT practice. They also prompted subsequent studies involving rigorous experimental designs and a diversity of clients, problems, and settings.

Later Studies and Research Reviews

The quantity and quality of SFT effectiveness studies and research reviews have increased steadily in recent decades. The first systematic review of SFT (Gingerich & Eisengart, 2000) included 15 studies conducted prior to 1999. Five were considered "well controlled" and nine "moderately or poorly controlled." Four of the five well-controlled studies showed positive outcomes, and the remaining nine supported the overall effectiveness of SFT.

Gingerich and Peterson (2013) conducted a qualitative review of 43 adequately controlled studies addressing various problems, settings, and clients from several different countries. Clients included children, adults, and couples experiencing a host of social, behavioral, and emotional problems. Of the 43 studies, 74% reported significant client benefits that included improvements in emotional health, behavioral functioning, and marital relationships; child and adolescent school problems; and other areas of social and psychological well-being. The authors concluded that there was solid evidence supporting the effectiveness of SFT for adults and young people experiencing a wide range of problems—with the added benefits of being more efficient and less costly than other treatments. Unlike the ultra-controlled laboratories and conditions of efficacy studies, SFT research is usually conducted in places where most therapists and clients typically meet—community mental health centers, clinics, private practice settings, and schools, to name a few.

A growing number of studies have employed randomized controlled trials (RCTs), often considered the gold standard for evaluating the effectiveness of a therapy approach. According to one list of evaluation studies on SFT, a total of 143 RCTs had been completed through March 2017 (Macdonald, 2017). The list indicated that SFT compared favorably with other approaches and that the average length of therapy was between 3 and 6.5 sessions per client. The number of RCTs exceeded 150 in 2021 (de Shazer et al., 2021), a number that is likely to rise steadily going forward.

The increasing number of RCTs and other well-designed studies has strengthened SFT's evidence base and encouraged large-scale reviews and meta-analyses of its impact or effect size for various problems and client populations. Meta-analyses of SFT studies have reported small overall effect sizes ranging from "very little" to "large" (Kim et al., 2019). These effect sizes are comparable with those reported in meta-analyses of other approaches based on studies conducted in natural, real-world settings. After examining eight meta-analyses of SFT studies involving a diversity of cultures, clients, and concerns, Kim et al. (2019) concluded that there was strong support for the wide-ranging effectiveness of SFT.

Research With Children and Adolescents

The bulk of psychotherapy outcome studies has involved adult clients, which makes sense given the extensive ethical and logistical requirements of clinical research with children and adolescents. The rapid increase in child and adolescent therapy clients highlights the importance of evaluating the effectiveness of contemporary therapy approaches with young clients. Fortunately, the number of well-designed studies of SFT with children and adolescents has increased steadily over the past 30 years.

The bulk of SFT research with young clients has occurred in schools because most child/adolescent referrals involve a school component, and SFT is particularly well suited to the realities of schools and school practitioners (Murphy, 2023). In one review, Kim (2008) reported that most school-based outcome studies have yielded small to medium effect sizes typical of those reported in community-based research of other therapy approaches with young people. Kim et al. (2017) reported similar findings, adding that SFT is a practical fit for school practitioners because it "is offered with only a few clinical sessions and has been shown to perform in a manner similar to other therapeutic approaches conducted in community settings with longer therapy sessions" (p. 45). A meta-analysis of solution-focused group therapy in schools indicated similarly positive effects (Gong & Hsu, 2017). Studies have shown individual and group SFT interventions to be effective in improving academic performance and grades (Sobhy & Cavallaro, 2010), school attendance and dropout rates (Franklin et al., 2018), internalizing problems (Gong & Hsu, 2017), and other social, behavioral, and psychological difficulties (Gong & Hsu, 2017; Kim et al., 2017).

Summary of Outcome Research on the Effectiveness of SFT

As with any therapy approach, there is a continued need for well-designed studies of SFT with a variety of clients, cultures, and difficulties. However, therapists and other practitioners can implement SFT with the assurance that it generally works as well as other approaches—and usually does so in fewer sessions.

Effectiveness studies help to establish the overall credibility and evidence base of a therapy approach as it compares with control and placebo treatments, other treatments, or no treatment. However, these studies provide limited information about how or why a particular approach is effective—not because they are flawed but because they are not designed to provide such information. There are two other sources of research that support SFT's effectiveness and shed light on how and why it works—process research and common factors research.

PROCESS RESEARCH ON SFT

Findings from microanalysis studies and other process research have clarified key processes and mechanisms of change in SFT, along with related differences between SFT and other approaches. *Microanalysis* is a qualitative research technique that examines therapeutic content and processes by analyzing minute segments of client–therapist communication (Bavelas, 2012). It is one of the most effective ways to link specific client–therapist interactions to broader processes, mechanisms of change, and patterns that characterize a therapy approach and distinguish it from other approaches. For example, client-directed solution talk in SFT has been verified in multiple microanalyses and linked to effective therapy outcomes (Beyebach, 2014; Franklin et al., 2017).

The purposeful use of language is central to SFT: "Our clients have taught us that solutions involve a very different kind of thinking and talking . . . that is . . . outside the problem" (Berg & de Shazer, 1993, p. 9). Comparative microanalyses have confirmed that solution-focused therapists refer to strengths and other positive aspects of clients' lives more than do cognitive behavior therapy (CBT) therapists (Froerer & Jordan, 2013; Smock Jordan et al., 2013) and that SFT sessions include more positive content from therapists and clients compared with CBT and motivational interviewing (MI) sessions (Korman et al., 2013; Smock Jordan et al., 2013).

Another language-related process that distinguishes SFT from other approaches is the therapist's use of the client's exact words in constructing therapy goals and follow-up questions. Microanalyses have confirmed that SFT therapists do this more often than therapists of other orientations. For example, Korman et al. (2013) found that SFT therapists used clients' specific words and phrases to coconstruct goals, ask questions, and build solutions more than cognitive behavior therapy (CBT) and motivational interviewing therapists. The researchers discovered another major difference between these approaches when it came to therapist "formulations." A *formulation* is a therapist comment that directly follows a client statement—often called a reflection or paraphrase. Korman et al. (2013) found that the formulations of solution-focused therapists, when compared with those of CBT and motivational interviewing therapists, included a higher percentage of clients' words and a lower percentage of interpretations.

In addition to preserving more of the client's language and key words, solution-focused therapists' formulations and questions included more references to productive aspects of clients' lives than the formulations and questions of CBT therapists (Smock Jordan et al., 2013). The same study reported that positive talk by therapists led to positive talk by clients and that negative therapist talk led to negative talk by clients. The above studies indicate that clients tend to respond in kind and follow therapists' lead when it comes to the content and focus of therapy conversations. In a large-scale microanalysis of the relationship between client outcomes and the content of therapy, Gassmann and Grawe (2006) found that the least successful therapists spent more time addressing client problems while the most successful ones spent more time discussing client strengths and resources—prompting the conclusion that therapy is most successful when clients experience themselves as more than the sum of their problems.

The microanalyses studies described above provide empirical support and clarification of the following SFT processes and practices: therapists' emphasis on exceptions, strengths, and other client resources; therapists' use of formulations and questions that incorporate the client's language; the coconstructive, solution-building impact of client–therapist dialogue; and the centralization of client language and preferences in the construction of therapeutic goals and solutions. In summary, process research has strengthened the evidence base of SFT by clarifying how and why it works.

COMMON FACTORS AND SFT

Drawing from decades of outcome studies and dozens of meta-analyses, psychotherapy researchers have concluded that successful outcomes result largely from the activation of several interrelated ingredients of therapy. These ingredients are called *common factors* (or nonspecific factors) because they are common to effective outcomes regardless of the practitioner's theoretical orientation or model (Norcross & Lambert, 2019).

The impact of common factors has been documented for nearly a century, beginning with Rosenzweig's classic article (1936) and continuing through the research of Frank and Frank (1991), Lambert (2013), and many others. Most of these investigations were conducted by career researchers with no allegiance to one therapy approach over another. The following discussion draws largely on the research and writings of

Lambert, Wampold, Norcross, Hill, and Duncan (Castonguay & Hill, 2017; Duncan, 2014; Norcross & Lambert, 2019; Wampold & Imel, 2015).

Five of the most powerful and well-researched common factors are *client, therapist, alliance, hope,* and *model/technique.* The success of any therapy approach depends largely on the extent to which it activates these potent elements of change. Common factors are fluid and interconnected rather than static and discrete, which is why the activation of one factor often activates the others. The interdependency of these elements makes it difficult to determine the exact impact of each one (Finsrud et al., 2022). However, researchers have identified the most powerful common factors, which are described next with attention to how they are addressed in SFT.

Client Factors

Client factors consist of everything the client brings to therapy to help them achieve their desired outcomes. This includes unique strengths, personal traits, and other resources such as clients' values, strengths, cultural customs, previous successes, special interests, spiritual beliefs/activities, social and community supports, and other aspects of the client's life that can help them achieve their therapy goals. Client factors are the most powerful of all common factors, accounting for a markedly larger portion of therapeutic change or outcome variance than any other aspect of therapy (Norcross & Lambert, 2019). It is not surprising that researchers have stated that "the time has come to set the story straight" and "to spotlight the largest and most neglected factor in treatment outcome: the client" (Bohart & Tallman, 2010, p. 84).

In contrast to the medical model's notion that therapists' interventions operate on clients to cure disorders and restore health, research indicates that clients adapt and use therapy techniques and conversations to produce positive outcomes (Bohart & Tallman, 2010; Murphy & Sparks, 2018). These findings confirm the fact that *all change is self-change,* regardless of whether it occurs with or without the help of therapy (Prochaska et al., 1994). Effective therapists help clients produce their own change by tailoring services to the client rather than requiring clients to conform to the therapist's perspectives and preferences (Norcross & Lambert, 2019).

Solution-focused therapists heed these findings by centralizing clients' input and resources throughout the therapy process, which includes involving them in setting the direction for therapy; building on exceptions and other cultural, social, and personal resources that they bring to therapy; asking how they have progressed and kept going in the face of significant challenges; requesting their feedback on the usefulness of therapy; and adjusting services based on their feedback and progress. Client factors are always there for the asking, and solution-focused therapists actively seek them out in every session.

Therapist Factors

Therapist factors, also called therapist effects, refer to the impact of the therapist on client outcomes beyond therapy models or techniques. Researchers have identified several attributes, abilities, and actions that distinguish the most effective therapists from others (Castonguay & Hill, 2017; Duncan, 2014; Norcross & Lambert, 2019). These include providing empathy, encouragement, and validation; respecting and honoring clients' worldviews; believing in clients' ability to improve their lives and in the efficacy of one's therapy approach in helping them do so; facilitating active client participation; forming collaborative alliances with a diversity of clients; tailoring services to client characteristics, culture, and preferences; collecting real-time client feedback; and spotlighting client strengths and resources. These evidence-based characteristics and actions fit well with SFT and are consistent with research and recommendations on culturally responsive therapy (D. W. Sue et al., 2019).

Clients' response to a therapy approach or technique may depend more on *who* delivers it than *what* it is (Wampold & Imel, 2015). The significance of therapist factors was dramatically illustrated in a large, federally funded research study on the treatment of depression that examined the relative effectiveness of antidepressant pills plus clinical management and placebo (sugar) pills plus clinical management (Elkin et al., 1989). Clients who received sugar pills from the top third or "most effective" psychiatrists had better outcomes than those who received antidepressants from the bottom third or "least effective" psychiatrists. Even in seemingly less personalized services such as medication prescription and management, the person who delivers the service makes a big difference in how clients respond to it.

Solution-focused therapists are responsive to the above findings by adopting a client-centered position of cultural humility; tailoring services to client preferences and goals rather than expecting or requiring clients to conform to therapist-driven goals and preferences; and requesting and honoring client input and feedback throughout the therapy process, including their input on when to schedule sessions and when to end therapy, as seen with Jalen and Rosa in Chapter 4. As Norcross and Lambert (2019) stated, therapist factors are "strong, ubiquitous, and sadly ignored in most guidelines on what works" (p. 8).

Research also suggests that strengths-based attitudes and activities on the part of therapists are more effective than deficit-based perspectives and actions. In the large-scale microanalysis study discussed earlier (Gassmann & Grawe, 2006), therapists who focused on clients' strengths and resources were more effective than those who focused on clients' problems and deficits. In another study involving 296 clients, researchers found that a "growing sense of self-esteem in the interaction with the therapist" was the strongest predictor of whether clients stayed in therapy or dropped out (Kegel & Flückiger, 2015, p. 383). Solution-focused therapists honor these findings by helping clients discover and build on exceptions, strengths, and other resources within themselves and their lives—a culturally responsive feature of SFT that may be particularly effective with clients from nondominant and underrepresented populations (Boyd-Franklin et al., 2013; Corey, 2023).

Alliance Factors

The therapeutic alliance or working relationship between the client and therapist consists of their interpersonal bond and their agreement on therapeutic goals, topics, and tasks (Bordin, 1979). The strength and quality of the alliance depend largely on the client's experience of respect, empathy, positive regard, validation, and encouragement from the therapist. These core conditions of effective therapeutic relationships—highlighted by Rogers (1957) over a half a century ago—have been consistently corroborated ever since (Norcross & Lambert, 2019).

Alliance factors influence therapy outcomes at a level similar to therapist factors (Wampold & Imel, 2015). The client's experience of the alliance is a reliable predictor of outcomes (Horvath et al., 2011; Norcross & Lambert, 2019) regardless of whether services are delivered online or in person (Flückiger et al., 2018). The early alliance is especially powerful. For example, several outcome studies have reported strong correlations between the client's perception of the alliance during the first few sessions (for better or worse) and the ultimate success or failure of therapy (Norcross & Lambert, 2019). SFT practitioners facilitate strong alliances by establishing a client-focused relationship and direction from the outset of services ("What are your best hopes from therapy?") and maintaining it by requesting ongoing client feedback on the effectiveness of services.

Hope (or Expectancy) Factors

Hope factors (hereafter "hope")—also called expectancy factors, outcome expectations, and placebo effects—consist of clients' anticipation of desired outcomes (expectancy) and confidence in their ability to achieve them (self-efficacy). The impact of hope on therapy outcomes is about the same as that of alliance and therapist factors, respectively (Norcross & Lambert, 2019). Some researchers have suggested that therapy models and techniques achieve their effects primarily through the activation of client hope (Hubble et al., 2010).

The activation of hope results partly from the well-documented placebo effect that was first noticed in drug research. The placebo effect occurs when people who receive a sham drug or *placebo*—a pill that looks just like the actual drug but lacks any active chemical ingredients—report feeling better than people who receive nothing and often as good as those who receive the drug. The placebo effect has been repeatedly verified in medicine and psychotherapy (Enck & Zipfel, 2019), suggesting that people who expect to get better usually do.

Self-efficacy, the belief in one's ability to achieve a specific goal, is another key component of hope. Hopeful clients expect to improve and attribute progress to *their* efforts and behavior. In multiple studies of self-efficacy, Dweck and Master (2008) reported that children who attributed achievements to their efforts and actions were more persistent and successful than those who attributed achievements to luck or chance. Solution-focused therapists capitalize on these findings by exploring the client's role in exceptions and progress ("How did you make it happen?" "What does that say about you?") and asking them to elaborate on their resilience and other attributes that have helped them overcome and cope with obstacles, setbacks, and other challenges ("How did you manage to push through and keep going?"). As seen with Trey in Chapter 1, sometimes one solution-focused question ("With everything you've been through, how do you keep hanging in there and coming to school?") and answer ("My aunt always tells me to never give up because quitters don't make it") can ignite a spark of hope that helps clients move forward and keep going.

Model/Technique Factors

Model/technique factors refer to the theoretical tenets and techniques that are unique to a specific therapy approach. Decades of empirical studies comparing different therapies across various clients and problems suggest that all evidence-based approaches are equally effective and that the impact of an approach's specific effects (technical differences between the approach and other approaches) is relatively small compared with its general effects (Finsrud et al., 2022; Wampold & Imel, 2015).

Given that everything we do in therapy can be seen as techniques and that common factors account for the largest portion of therapeutic change, it is useful to consider how therapy models and techniques influence outcomes. Researchers offer two answers. First, models and techniques provide needed structure and consistency for clients as well as therapists (Wampold & Imel, 2015). Second, techniques achieve their effects largely through their activation of client resources, hope, involvement, and other common factors (Hubble et al., 2010; Wampold & Imel, 2015). In other words, techniques serve as conduits through which other common factors are activated.

The relatively small impact of model/technique factors does not mean they are unimportant. Everything a therapist does is a technique of one kind or another, and techniques are based on a therapeutic rationale or theory of change. The most effective therapists apply their theoretical and technical expertise in ways that optimize client factors, hope, alliance, and other common factors of change.

Summary of Common Factors Research and SFT

As noted throughout this discussion, SFT activates the powerful common factors of therapeutic change in many distinct and specific ways—an added source of empirical integrity for SFT. To be clear, all established therapies activate common factors to one extent or another. However, the collaborative and strengths-based elements of SFT make it particularly responsive to these factors.

After reviewing several outcome studies on change factors in SFT, Beyebach (2014) stated, "Seen from a 'common factors' perspective . . . solution focused therapy provides a dialogical process that allows therapeutic common factors to emerge to their best advantage" and that "solution-focused conversational practices might promote in very specific and intentional ways the therapeutic factors that too often are considered unspecific or beyond the influence of the therapist" (p. 72). Kort et al. (2021) provided additional information on the complementary nature of solution-focused practice and common factors and on the clinical advantages of adopting a "common factors perspective" of SFT as reflected in this book.

TRANSCULTURAL EVALUATION OF SFT

This section offers evidence of SFT's transcultural effectiveness along with possible reasons why it is effective with clients from many different backgrounds, cultures, and countries. The international use of SFT has rapidly grown in recent decades, as has outcome research on its impact with an increasingly wide range of clients on every continent (Beyebach et al., 2021). This research includes RCTs, meta-analyses, and quasi-experimental outcome studies conducted with clients of various ethnicities and countries. A few representative studies of SFT's transcultural effectiveness, including studies involving clients from underrepresented groups, are described next.

One of the first studies to examine the impact of SFT with clients from underrepresented populations was conducted at the Brief Family Therapy Center in Milwaukee (De Jong & Hopwood, 1996). This study examined intermediate and final outcome data of 275 clients over the course of 2 years. Clients included children, adolescents, and adults—57% identified as African Americans, 5% as Latinx, and 36% as White; 43% of the adults were employed when they began therapy and 57% were unemployed. Self-reported outcome data from clients were compared across race, age, gender, and employment status. Clients showed minimal differences in intermediate and final outcomes across all demographic categories, which led researchers to suggest that SFT appeared to be effective with a diversity of client populations. Of the 137 clients who responded to a follow-up survey 7 to 9 months after therapy ended, 72% reported satisfaction with their services, 16% said they were neither satisfied nor dissatisfied, and 12% were dissatisfied. Researchers found no major differences in client satisfaction across race, age, gender, or employment status.

Although the earliest writings and research on SFT occurred in the United States and Europe, empirical evaluation of SFT now includes many other countries. After examining 365 outcome studies from numerous countries, Beyebach et al. (2021) reported that (a) outcome research on SFT has rapidly increased in recent decades, (b) the number of studies in nonindustrialized countries outside the United States and Europe has grown significantly, (c) the quality of SFT research has become consistently stronger (as evidenced in part by the fact that almost half of the studies reviewed were RCTs), and (d) the results of their review confirmed the broad applicability and effectiveness of SFT as the sole or main intervention for a diverse range of problems and client groups throughout the world. In a follow-up review of 251 outcome studies, Neipp and Beyebach

(2022) similarly concluded that SFT "is demonstrating effectiveness transculturally, for a variety of practices (psychotherapy, coaching, school counseling, etc.) and intervention formats (individual, group, family/couples)" (p. 15).

Empirical research on SFT with Chinese clients provides an example of the approach's growing evidence base with non-Western clients and countries. In a meta-analysis of nine studies completed in China, Kim et al. (2015) reported that SFT was effective in helping Chinese clients reduce a variety of internalizing problems and other mental health challenges. Gong and Xu (2015) completed a meta-analysis of 33 studies of SFT with child and adult Chinese clients and concluded that SFT was an effective approach with clients experiencing a wide array of behavioral and psychological difficulties. Gong and Hsu (2017) came to a similar conclusion based on a meta-analysis involving 24 experimental and quasi-experimental studies of solution-focused group therapy with Chinese school students.

These are just a few of the many empirical studies, reviews, and meta-analyses that have verified the effectiveness of SFT with a diversity of clients, problems, and cultures throughout the world—including clients from underrepresented and underserved racial/ethnic groups and intersectional identities.

Possible Reasons for SFT's Transcultural Effectiveness

There are many possible reasons why SFT works with underrepresented clients and clients from different cultures and countries. SFT is a client-directed approach in which client opinions, preferences, and perceptions take precedence over those of the therapist. Therapists encourage clients to establish the goal of therapy and apply their indigenous resources toward achieving it. Clients from nondominant groups may respond particularly well to being asked their opinions and being recognized for the resources they bring to therapy. Jalen, the African American client from Chapter 4, reinforced this point when he told the therapist, "It's nice to be asked your opinion of things. Nobody asks me what I think about things, they usually just tell me what I should be doing or not doing. I've heard that all my life."

Jalen's comment helps to explain why SFT works with underrepresented clients and why therapist-dominated approaches have been largely unsuccessful for this population (S. Sue & Zane, 2006).

Centralizing the client's goals and resources is a core feature of SFT, as is the therapist's awareness of the adverse effects that certain sociocultural messages, injustices, and experiences can have on underrepresented clients. Rather than diagnosing, blaming, or otherwise telling clients what is wrong with them and what they (in Jalen's words) "should be doing or not doing," SFT therapists acknowledge their problems and ask what they want instead. These strengths-based elements of SFT enhance its transcultural effectiveness and distinguish it from deficit-based approaches in which therapists diagnose clients and prescribe interventions.

Acknowledging clients' resources and inviting them to apply these assets toward desired outcomes can also boost minority clients' sense of hope, possibility, and self-efficacy—which may in turn help them push through obstacles and persist in their journey to a better future (Dweck, 2016). Multicultural researchers have consistently recommended strengths-based therapy approaches for clients from underrepresented racial and ethnic populations (D. W. Sue et al., 2019). For example, Boyd-Franklin et al. (2013) urged therapists to use strengths-focused methods with African American clients, who are often more aware of their problems than their strengths. One of the most obvious ways SFT therapists do this is by helping clients identify and build on exceptions and other strengths that support desired outcomes.

The radically client-directed focus of SFT is another possible reason why it has been effective with clients from nondominant cultures and backgrounds (Corey, 2023). In contrast to approaches in which the therapist selects therapy goals and prescribes interventions for achieving them, solution-focused therapists invite clients to apply their resources toward self-selected goals. Although these features apply to all clients, their impact may be strongest for those from underrepresented racial/ethnic groups who enter services "feeling powerless" and "gain a sense of empowerment and ownership . . . when they participate in their own goal setting" (Ridley, 2005, p. 107). Giving clients a central voice in every aspect of their care enhances their investment in services and ownership of therapy gains, both of which are keys to culturally responsive, socially just services (Crethar et al., 2008; D. W. Sue et al., 2019).

The collaborative and empowering elements of SFT have also been reported by clients. In a recent study (Zak, 2022) involving 346 SFT clients from Poland (ages 18–67; 74% female), clients were asked what aspects of therapy were most helpful to them. Clients reported beneficial effects of being heard and understood, becoming aware of their personal strengths, the therapist's faith in their ability to change, and the therapist's confirmation of what they were doing right. As one client put it: "For me, it was helpful that you encouraged me to think without giving advice to 'do this or that' because this is a difficult situation . . ." (p. 14). Although the race and ethnicity of this client are unknown, their words mirror the experience of Jalen and other clients from nondominant backgrounds and cultural groups.

CRITICISMS AND POTENTIAL DISADVANTAGES

The following potential disadvantages and criticisms of SFT occasionally come up in classes and workshops, online discussion groups, and psychotherapy textbooks.

Potential Disadvantages

Many of the potential disadvantages described below are the very things about the SFT approach that appeal to solution-focused practitioners and their clients.

Simple but Not Easy

SFT is simple but not easy—simple to describe but hard to master. Implementing SFT requires extensive discipline, focus, and faith in clients' capabilities. Although conceptual simplicity is one of SFT's most appealing features, it has led some practitioners to assume that it is easier to master than other approaches. This misunderstanding may result in a practitioner's overemphasizing techniques at the expense of closely attending to what clients say, echoing their words in follow-up questions, and addressing other nuances of solution-focused work. Corey (2023) observed that practitioners with an incomplete or superficial knowledge of SFT may glorify solution-focused techniques and view them as ends in themselves— a tendency frequently observed among graduate students and practitioners new to the approach. For example, a novice practitioner might simply ask the miracle question without following up on the client's response to elicit a more detailed solution description.

As Lipchik (2002) noted, SFT requires therapists go "beyond technique" by acknowledging clients' emotions, picking up on verbal and nonverbal client nuances and cues, and maintaining strong therapeutic alliances. As with any therapy approach, mastering SFT requires rigorous training, practice, and supervision—along with regular reminders that it is simple to understand but far from easy to implement.

Descriptive and Client-Directed
(vs. Interpretive and Therapist-Directed)

For over a century, psychotherapists interpreted the underlying meanings and motives of client actions, feelings, and comments. In contrast, solution-focused therapists accept client comments at face value instead of trying to interpret or explain them. They also stay "close to the surface" by formulating follow-up questions from clients' previous answers and trusting clients to translate therapeutic conversations into workable solutions.

With the above points in mind, SFT's emphasis on centralizing the client and decentralizing the therapist may not be a good fit for clients who want a therapist to interpret their problems and tell them how to resolve them. These clients might be better served by a more authoritarian, psychodynamic approach. However, clients who enter therapy expecting to learn more about their problem may be open to trying SFT for a session or two before deciding whether to stay with it or try something different. The descriptive and client-directed features of SFT may pose other possible disadvantages for therapists as noted below.

Colleagues May Not Be Impressed. Because SFT downplays the cleverness of the therapist and therapist interventions, colleagues may be unimpressed by the approach and the therapists who use it. They may view the approach as overly simplistic, naïve, and trustful of clients as reflected in questions such as, "If clients already have the resources needed to change their lives, then why would they be in therapy?" or "How can just talking with clients help them change?" SFT may not be a good fit for therapists who raise these questions and concerns.

The potential disadvantage of SFT's straightforward approach was dramatically illustrated during a supervision session with Devon,[1] a doctoral student who had been using SFT for about a year. Even though most of his clients had achieved successful outcomes, Devon expressed the following concern: "SFT usually works, but it's so plain that I don't feel like a *real* therapist doing *real* therapy." He added that his case reviews at weekly staff meetings were shorter and less intriguing than those of other practitioners from different theoretical orientations. The supervisor acknowledged Devon's concerns and asked him, "What is the goal of therapy?" Devon smiled and replied, "To help clients achieve *their* goals, not mine." He is currently a practicing solution-focused therapist.

Requires Restraint and Discipline. Being client directed does not come naturally for many therapists, perhaps because of the professional pressure for therapists to offer clever solutions to people's problems. Solution-focused therapists resist the urge to give advice and accept the client's goals instead of steering them toward therapist-driven goals. This type of discipline and restraint is a lot harder than it sounds. For example, it may be difficult for a therapist to accept the client's goal of improving their marriage when the therapist thinks they should work through their childhood trauma experiences. The same holds true when clients say they have achieved their goals and want to end therapy when the therapist thinks they should continue. These examples illustrate the challenge of keeping one's ideas to oneself in favor of asking questions that invite clients to develop their own solutions.

Clients Are Responsible for Successes but Not Failures. Another possible drawback of SFT for practitioners is that when therapy is successful, the client gets the credit; when therapy fails, it is the therapist's responsibility

---

[1] Identifying details for all individuals in this example have been removed for confidentiality purposes.

to adjust services to better fit the client. Solution-focused therapists do not view therapeutic failures as signs of client resistance, lack of motivation, or other such things. Instead, they assume responsibility for finding different ways to be more useful to the client. This perspective is difficult to implement and hard on the therapist's ego.

Psychotherapy Is a Problem-Focused Profession. The psychotherapy profession is steeped in problem-focused traditions that embrace clinical diagnosis and prescriptive interventions—both of which are antithetical to SFT. This can make it difficult for some therapists to move from a problem-based approach to a solution-focused approach. Despite the growing evidence base and popularity of SFT, solution-focused therapists may be the only practitioners in their agencies who are using SFT. Although this can make it lonely and isolating for solution-focused therapists, many practitioners in these situations have received support from in-person or online discussion groups, blogs, listservs, and other sources of connection and collaboration with solution-focused colleagues. They have also benefitted from reminding themselves why they were attracted to SFT in the first place—privileging clients' goals versus practitioners' goals, focusing on future possibilities versus past problems, and other differences between solution-focused and problem-focused practice.

Logistical Challenges. In contrast to the long-standing therapeutic tradition of seeing clients every week, SFT often involves longer intervals between sessions depending on the client's preference, progress, and other client-driven considerations. It also involves ending therapy when clients say they have reached their goals, regardless of how many sessions that may be. These client-centered aspects of SFT may pose scheduling, financial, and other logistical challenges for some practitioners and agencies.

Potential Misuse. All therapy approaches are subject to practitioner misuse, and SFT is no exception. There are innumerable ways any approach can be misused, and the following discussion describes a few common misuses of SFT.

One of the biggest challenges for therapists who adopt an approach that appeals to them and works for most of their clients is doing something different when it doesn't work for a client. Although it is helpful to be enthusiastic about one's therapy approach, unbridled loyalty to SFT in the absence of client benefit contradicts the approach's client-driven philosophy and "do something different" guideline. The longer a therapist uses an approach, the less likely they may be to abandon it when clients are not benefiting.

Although SFT's brevity appeals to many therapists, the approach can be misused when they overemphasize brevity at the expense of client preferences and outcomes. For example, practitioners may directly or indirectly pressure clients into ending therapy before they have achieved their goals and are ready to end services. An overzealous SFT clinician might minimize the complexities of a client's situation to sustain their record and reputation as a brief therapist. Sometimes "less and simpler" is not better for certain clients, which highlights the importance of obtaining ongoing client feedback on the usefulness and fit of SFT services (Gillaspy & Murphy, 2012). de Shazer (as cited in Ratner et al., 2012) advocated for therapeutic efficiency but avoided defining "brief" as a certain number of sessions—preferring instead to say therapy should last as long as it takes and not one session more. The subtext of this comment is that the number of sessions—and all other decisions in SFT—should emerge from close collaboration with the client.

Criticisms

SFT has mistakenly been characterized as ignoring problems and emotions, not working for serious problems, being mechanistic and solution-forced, and being too trustful of clients.

SFT Ignores Problems

The most common criticism and misconception about SFT is that it is overly positive and thus ignores problems and prevents clients from talking about them. This criticism usually results from a superficial understanding of SFT or a lack of opportunity to see it in action. First, SFT is about being useful rather than positive. Second, solution-focused therapists neither ignore problems nor prevent clients from discussing them—to do so would be unwise and disrespectful given that problems are what bring clients to therapy in the first place.

Solution-focused therapists fully acknowledge problems and provide space for clients to discuss them. As de Shazer et al. (2021) noted, "creating a space for or 'honoring' the problem is vital to therapy if clients are to feel that the therapist understands their predicament and is interested in helping" (p. 153). The client's experience of being listened to and understood is an essential part of effective alliances and outcomes (Elliott et al., 2019), and listening is the foundation of all other therapist activities and techniques in SFT.

Besides its name, one explanation for the misconception that SFT ignores problems—and one of the biggest differences between SFT and problem-focused approaches—pertains to what happens *after* the therapist acknowledges the client's problem. Whereas problem-focused therapists follow up by exploring problem-related history and details, SFT therapists ask what clients want instead.

SFT Ignores Emotions

SFT also has been criticized as ignoring clients' emotions. It is true that solution-focused therapists ask fewer questions about client emotions than do other therapists. For example, it is unlikely for a therapist to ask, "Why do you think you felt that way?" because it would not lead to a fuller description of the client's preferred future or progress toward it. However, solution-focused therapists validate clients' feelings whenever they arise during therapy sessions ("That sounds awful," "No wonder you felt so bad"). They also accept client goals that include feelings ("I want to feel happier, more energetic, etc.") and invite clients to describe additional actions, thoughts, social interactions, and other details of their preferred future associated with feeling happier or more energetic.

Although solution-focused therapists acknowledge and validate clients' feelings, they do not explore them in great depth. Instead of focusing on feelings per se, therapists believe that "situating emotional states in outward actions and contexts is more useful" (de Shazer et al., 2021, p. 154) because those are the contexts of greatest concern and significance for most clients. Questions might include "What will you be doing differently when you're happier? How will your family respond?" and "What would that be like for you?" These questions also reflect SFT's interest in the client's description of life "outside of the therapy session," which differentiates SFT from approaches that focus on what clients are feeling and experiencing in the session itself. Since client concerns and solutions occur *outside* of therapy, SFT focuses on what is happening for clients outside rather than inside the therapy room.

SFT Can Be Mechanistic and Solution-Forced

This criticism has more to do with *who* is implementing SFT than with the approach itself. Any therapy approach can become mechanistic and less effective when the therapist loses sight of the person across from them and becomes overly focused on techniques. In SFT, this may occur when therapists pressure clients into identifying exceptions, reporting positive improvements, or anything else that replaces client-directed/solution-focused practice with therapist-directed/solution-forced practice. Nylund and Corsiglia (1994) used the phrase "solution-forced therapy" to describe what can happen when therapists misuse SFT in these ways—which is why SFT trainers caution students and practitioners about these and other solution-forced actions that compromise the integrity and effectiveness of SFT. As any SFT practitioner or trainer can attest, SFT is deceptively simple to describe but far from easy to implement.

SFT Does Not Work for Serious Problems

SFT is sometimes perceived as a band-aid approach that is effective for mild problems but not serious ones. This misperception is often based on superficial impressions of the approach as reflected in questions such as, "How can you help clients without exploring the root of their problems?" or "How can 'just talking' help someone manage trauma and other serious problems?"

These questions are closely related to another one that comes up in classes and workshops: "How does SFT work with this-or-that type of problem or client?" The question itself implies that it is possible to know how a therapy approach will work before using it with a client. It is not, which is why it is so important to obtain client feedback and adjust one's approach when it is not helping the client. A partial answer to this question can be found in studies and meta-analyses supporting SFT's overall effectiveness with broad categories of clients and difficulties. For example, SFT has been effective with children, adults, couples, and families who experience depression, anxiety, and relationship problems. It has also proven effective with clients in long-term care (Simon & Nelson, 2007) and persons experiencing trauma (Froerer et al., 2018), schizophrenia (Panayotov et al., 2012), self-harming (Selekman, 2009), and other serious problems.

Given increased public and professional attention to the topic of trauma and its treatment, it is not surprising that several "trauma-informed" therapies have recently emerged. A thorough review of empirical studies and meta-analyses reported that specifically designated trauma-informed or trauma-focused therapies were no more effective than other established approaches with clients who have experienced trauma (Norcross & Wampold, 2019). The researchers explained this finding by highlighting the substantial impact of client and therapist factors, the therapeutic alliance, and other common factors of change—all of which are supported and activated by SFT.

The inaccurate criticism that SFT does not work for serious problems may also reflect the perception that solution-focused conversations lack proper depth because they stay "on the surface" of clients' answers rather going deeper and interpreting their underlying meaning. This criticism reflects three unproven assumptions of traditional psychotherapy. First, client statements cannot be trusted at face value. Second, problems are symptoms of deeper issues that fall outside of the client's awareness. Third, effective therapy requires diagnosing and treating the underlying causes of problems.

In contrast to the problem-focused, depth-based assumptions of traditional psychotherapy, SFT proposes that clients who experience serious problems can make effective and lasting changes by replacing problem-focused descriptions of themselves and their lives with detailed, solution-focused descriptions of their preferred futures—and by living in ways that support those futures. These propositions are supported by substantial evidence for the effectiveness of SFT with a variety of clients, cultures, and problems. This discussion is not meant to disparage depth-oriented approaches or to suggest that SFT is better or more effective than these or other established approaches. As de Shazer et al. (2021) pointed out, the perceived "depth" of a therapy approach depends on one's definition of depth. For example, although SFT does not explore client problems in great depth, it elicits wide and deep descriptions of what they want instead.

SFT Is Too Trustful of Clients

SFT has been criticized for placing too much trust in clients' capabilities by giving them a central voice in constructing goals, evaluating therapy, deciding when to end services, and other key aspects of their care. The implicit (and sometimes explicit) subtext of this critique is captured in the question "Are clients capable of knowing what is best for themselves?" This question reflects the patriarchal insinuations of the medical/disease model in which weak, sick "patients" are healed by expert doctors and treatments. The fact that Freud and most other psychotherapists of the late 19th and early 20th centuries were steeped in the medical model helps to clarify the origin of this question.

The main reason SFT has been criticized for being too trustful of clients is because it challenges the diagnostic/prescriptive model of psychiatry and psychotherapy that has prevailed for over 100 years. However, psychotherapy research over the past 50 years indicates that therapy outcomes depend largely on the extent to which clients are centralized and included in all major aspects their care (Duncan, 2014; Norcross & Lambert, 2019). This research encourages therapists to invite clients to collaborate on key decisions (Tryon et al., 2019), evaluate the usefulness of services (Lambert et al., 2019), and apply their indigenous resources toward desired outcomes (Bohart & Tallman, 2010; Duncan, 2014)—all of which are central to SFT.

REJOINDER TO CRITICISMS AND POTENTIAL DISADVANTAGES

Many of the alleged disadvantages and criticisms of SFT have resulted from limited familiarity with the approach and its evidence base, transcultural effectiveness, and clinical history. However, there are other reasons why it is taken longer for SFT to gain wider acceptance and legitimacy within the psychotherapy profession compared to other established approaches— including approaches with far less empirical support than SFT.

The main reason why the psychotherapy profession has been slow to embrace SFT is because its postmodern tenets and techniques challenge many modernist, Western-based assumptions and practices that have dominated the profession for over a century. For example, the medical-based practice of diagnosing clients and prescribing treatments is antithetical to SFT's view of clients as stuck versus sick and resourceful versus dependent on therapist-directed interventions. The modernist notion that a client's problem can be objectively defined and treated by a therapist-driven intervention contrasts with SFT's postmodern, social constructionist notion that most client problems and solutions are constructions created primarily by language, dialogue, and other forms of social interaction and meaning making. These ideas were met with skepticism and disdain when they were introduced in the psychotherapy literature by social constructionism theorists (McNamee & Gergen, 1992) and postmodern therapists associated with SFT (de Shazer, 1985), narrative therapy (White & Epston, 1990) and collaborative language systems therapy (H. Anderson & Goolishian, 1992). Postmodern ideas and methods have become increasingly valued and appreciated within the psychotherapy profession (Corey, 2023), as have postmodern therapies such as SFT.

Although SFT's efficiency is very appealing to clients, it has hindered its path to credibility in the psychotherapy profession. The idea that therapy can be effective in a few sessions, or even one, challenges the unproven belief among many therapists that "more is better" when it comes to the duration and depth of a therapy approach. This belief has persisted despite research indicating that most therapists engage in brief therapy whether they want to or not (Levenson, 2017), as discussed in Chapter 1. Research also confirms that the bulk of client change occurs during the first few sessions and there is a point of diminishing returns after that (Duncan, 2014; Hansen & Lambert, 2003). The fact that SFT is brief by design versus default honors these research findings as well as client preferences for less versus more when it comes to the length of therapy.

The conceptual simplicity and minimalism of SFT have also hindered its credibility by challenging time-honored therapy traditions and practices. For example, beginning therapy by simply asking clients what they want from it is a far cry from the elaborate intake interviews and diagnostic assessments that are standard first steps in other approaches. Encouraging clients to create self-selected goals and increase what they are already doing toward achieving them strikes many therapists as "too simple" to be effective. The solution-focused idea that having clients describe their goals in rich detail promotes therapeutic solutions seems too good to be true—and yet it is true for many SFT clients based on the empirical evidence.

SFT's journey to legitimacy has also been hampered by the limited and pragmatic focus of its theory—and by the misconception that it has no theory. Chapter 3 dispelled this misconception by describing how theory has always informed the development and practice of SFT. However, the unconventional nature of SFT theory differs markedly from traditional theories in that it focuses exclusively on what therapists and clients do together *in therapy sessions* that makes therapy successful. Unlike most psychotherapy theories, which were deduced from existing theories of personality and psychopathology, SFT theory makes no claims about why clients have problems or what solutions should look like. The inductive, evidence-based process by which SFT theory was constructed is one of its most unique and distinguishing features (Trepper & Franklin, 2012). This and other differences between SFT and traditional approaches help to explain why it has taken a relatively long time for SFT to gain the respect and appreciation it currently has within the psychotherapy profession.

SUMMARY

Decades of empirical research indicate that SFT is an evidence-based, transcultural approach that works as well as other approaches and generally does so in fewer sessions. The approach's practicality, cultural responsiveness, and proven effectiveness have solidified its standing in the psychotherapy profession and led to its regular inclusion as a postmodern approach in psychotherapy and counseling textbooks. The centralization of client goals, preferences, strengths, and feedback empowers common factors of therapeutic change and makes SFT particularly suitable for underrepresented clients from many countries, racial/ethnic backgrounds, and intersectional identities. Criticisms and disadvantages attributed to SFT have resulted largely from misunderstandings of the approach and major differences between SFT and traditional psychotherapies. Many of the alleged disadvantages and criticisms of SFT pertain to the very things practitioners and clients find most appealing about the approach.

6

Suggestions for Future Developments

This chapter offers hopes and suggestions for future developments in solution-focused therapy (SFT) research, practice, and training. These three areas are interdependent in that advances in one area can prompt developments in the others.

RESEARCH

Research and evidence-based practice have played a key role in SFT and will continue to do so in the future. The following suggestions are offered to enhance SFT research and promote an effective interplay between solution-focused research, practice, and training.

Sustain and Expand Effectiveness Research

The bulk of SFT research falls into the category of effectiveness research. In contrast to efficacy studies that assess the impact of treatment under

https://doi.org/10.1037/0000370-006
Solution-Focused Therapy, by J. J. Murphy

ideal and controlled circumstances, effectiveness studies are conducted in the real-world settings where most therapists work. Both approaches have their pros and cons when it comes to internal validity (the degree to which client changes are linked to treatment), external validity (the extent to which a study's results can be generalized to other contexts and clients), and the practicality of delivering the treatment as described.

Although efficacy studies have their place, effectiveness studies will likely remain the primary empirical means by which SFT is evaluated and refined going forward. For example, there has been a recent increase of SFT effectiveness studies that employ randomized designs in community mental health settings, family service clinics, hospitals, and other real-world settings. By balancing methodological rigor with the practical realities of clinical work, these studies hold great promise for assessing and informing SFT in the future.

There are also indications that future SFT research will encompass a progressively wider range of clients, countries, cultures, challenges, and contexts. For example, studies examined in the Kim et al. (2019) meta-analysis involved a diversity of nations and populations, including Chinese, Korean, North American, European, Latinx, and African American clients. The worldwide growth of SFT will encourage more effectiveness studies and meta-analyses involving a diversity of clients and cultures—a trend that is well underway according to Beyebach et al. (2021), who reported that SFT outcome studies have been completed in 33 countries from all continents.

Solution-focused practices have been increasingly applied in non-therapy contexts such as business, education, community planning, and many others. Although prior SFT research has targeted the therapy setting and will continue to do so in the future, the potential of solution-focused practice will be more fully realized when future studies examine its effectiveness in these and other promising contexts.

Conduct Research Reviews and Meta-Analyses

In addition to assessing the overall impact of SFT across many clients and problems, meta-analyses and research reviews clarify SFT's effectiveness with specific client populations, settings, and cultures. This can be helpful to policy makers and practitioners who work in these contexts. For example, school practitioners from China can take comfort in a recent meta-analysis that verified the effectiveness of SFT groups in Chinese schools (Gong & Hsu, 2017). The authors discussed the following possible reasons why SFT is effective with Chinese clients: SFT respects the client's choice of what to talk about in therapy, which fits well with the importance of "saving face" in Chinese culture; SFT focuses on strengths and resources versus weaknesses and deficiencies, which also fits with saving face; and SFT explores the role of family and significant others in the client's life, which honors the importance of relationships and interdependency in Chinese culture.

Encourage Practitioner Research

The increase in RCTs and sophisticated statistical analyses in SFT research has strengthened the approach's credibility as an evidence-based therapy. Although randomized designs and statistical analyses are familiar topics for professional researchers, most practitioners have neither the time nor inclination to engage in labor-intensive research activities on top of their daily clinical responsibilities. However, there are practical ways that solution-focused therapists can integrate research into their everyday duties. Therapists and agencies can collect session-by-session client feedback on outcome and alliance and use this practice-based evidence to adjust services and improve their overall effectiveness as service providers (Duncan, 2014). Routine outcome management systems such as the Partners for Change Outcome Management System (Duncan & Sparks, 2018) offer therapists and agencies evidence-based methods for applying the scientist–practitioner model on an ongoing basis.

Use Microanalysis to Examine SFT Processes

Microanalysis research analyzes minute segments of client–therapist interactions to better understand how language and communication works in SFT. Solution-focused theory proposes that dialogue is the primary means by which clients and therapists coconstruct new meanings and solutions in SFT. Future microanalyses will further clarify SFT processes and their impact on client outcomes.

Include Client Input and Perceptions

In keeping with the client-directed focus of SFT, future studies could include client input and perspectives in the design, implementation, and interpretation of research. This could be as simple as asking clients what was most and least helpful about their therapy experience or how they perceived specific questions or question sequences. Anecdotal information of this nature adds a useful qualitative element to other research data collected in effectiveness studies and other investigations of SFT.

Examine Cultural Influences

Even though SFT has been shown to be effective with clients from many different cultures and countries, there is much to be learned about the role and influence of cultural factors in SFT. This may involve examining (a) the impact of client–therapist cultural differences on outcomes, (b) how clients of different cultures experience specific SFT techniques, and (c) other culture-related questions and topics. The more therapists know about cultural influences, the more effective they will be with future clients.

PRACTICE

The need for mental health services has rapidly increased since the onset of the COVID-19 pandemic (Terlizzi & Schiller, 2022), and SFT is poised to address this need. Some clients can't or won't commit to long-term therapy, for personal, financial, logistical, or other reasons. This becomes a social justice issue when the availability of SFT or other short-term services is the difference between a person receiving or not receiving services.

The client-centered focus of SFT also increases the likelihood of offering socially just services across many cultures and underrepresented client populations. SFT encourages clients to establish self-selected goals, apply indigenous resources toward solutions, and provide ongoing feedback on the usefulness and fit of services. These and other aspects of SFT strengthen clients' ownership of successful outcomes and ensure socially just, culturally responsive services. The following suggestions are offered in the hopes of enhancing the future evolution, usefulness, and reach of SFT.

Adopt a Multicultural Orientation

Regardless of one's theoretical orientation, appreciating and accommodating cultural factors and cultural diversity is essential to one's effectiveness. This includes an awareness of how differences between a client's and therapist's worldviews, backgrounds, race, and other culture-loaded factors can impact power dynamics, communication styles, intervention preferences, and other key aspects of therapy.

Solution-focused therapists and their clients will continue to benefit from the therapist's cultural humility and adoption of a multicultural orientation as described in Chapter 3. Approaching every client as a culture of one and every session as a cross-cultural exchange reduces the likelihood of typecasting clients based on their diagnosis, ethnicity, gender, sexual orientation, or other narrow descriptions of clients and their lives.

Link Future Developments to Core Tenets

The more popular a therapy approach becomes, the more likely it is that it will be misunderstood and misused by people with limited knowledge of it. This has certainly been the case with SFT, as seen in Chapter 5's discussion of alleged disadvantages and criticisms of the approach. These misunderstandings and misuses highlight the importance of accurately describing SFT to others and linking future solution-focused developments to the approach's core tenets.

Adopt a Scientist–Practitioner Approach

The future of SFT depends partly on the extent to which individual practitioners (and the SFT community as a whole) adopt a scientist–practitioner model of clinical practice and development. There are many practical ways therapists can measure their effectiveness with individual clients, client groups, types of problems, and other aspects of practice. As noted earlier, therapists who regularly use the Outcome Rating Scale (Miller & Duncan, 2000) and Session Rating Scale (Miller et al., 2002) have a continuous supply of progress and alliance data they can use to improve their effectiveness and outcomes. The SFT community as a whole—which includes individual practitioners, professional organizations, training and certification programs, researchers, teachers and trainers, authors, and others—can promote the importance of scientific research in the future development and practice of SFT. The next suggestion addresses another key part of a scientist–practitioner approach to clinical work.

Stay Current

This suggestion is much easier said than done. Staying current on relevant research findings and practices in SFT, and psychotherapy in general, is essential to one's development and growth as an SFT practitioner. In addition to maintaining updated knowledge of new discoveries and developments in SFT, therapists (and their clients) will benefit from keeping abreast of important findings from psychotherapy research on common factors and other relevant topics.

Connect With Colleagues, Organizations, and Other Resources

Although there are benefits to having instant access to information about everything under the sun—including the ever-growing number of therapy approaches, techniques, and research findings—it can also impede a practitioner's development of sufficient expertise and depth in SFT. This is one of several reasons why it is useful to maintain regular connections and interactions with solution-focused colleagues. This can be done by participating in SFT discussion lists, podcasts, webinars, professional associations, conferences, and local or regional consultation groups.

Put Technology to Work

Advances in technology have created efficient, cost-effective ways to serve clients beyond traditional in-person meetings. Examples include text messaging, email, apps, and teletherapy sessions. Although many therapists and clients prefer in-person meetings to teletherapy sessions conducted online or by phone, new technologies have enabled therapists to serve more clients—many of whom are unable to access in-person services for economic, geographical, and other reasons. Research suggests that teletherapy and other online services are just as effective as in-person services (Andrews et al., 2018), which provides another reason for therapists to incorporate telecommunication strategies in their clinical practice.

Never Lose a Holy Curiosity

Physicist Albert Einstein urged people to "never lose a holy curiosity," which captures the attitude of SFT practitioners toward clients and the work of therapy. Rather than trying to interpret or explain people's difficulties and motives, therapists approach clients with respectful curiosity (Murphy & Sparks, 2018) and a sense of wonder and appreciation for their ability to keep going in the face of major life challenges. Solution-focused therapists embrace a similar sense of wonder for the work itself and the transformative quality of client–therapist dialogue. With these points in mind, solution-focused (and other) therapists have much to gain from heeding Einstein's advice to never lose a holy curiosity.

TRAINING

The following suggestions are offered in the hopes of enhancing the quality and usefulness of future training in SFT.

Walk the Walk

If you have ever experienced a "do as I say, not as I do" situation in which a supervisor's or trainer's actions contradicted their instruction, then you can appreciate the importance of delivering SFT training and supervision services in ways that reflect the approach's core tenets and techniques. To do otherwise compromises the benefits and outcomes of SFT training. For example, if a trainer or supervisor stresses the importance of listening in SFT while failing to properly listen and respond to trainees' questions, they are jeopardizing their credibility as well as the credibility and impact of what they are teaching.

SFT trainers "walk the walk" by adopting a solution-focused approach to training. They acknowledge that training is different from therapy and that certain aspects of SFT—for example, adopting a position of "not knowing" or not providing explanations—are not always appropriate in a training or supervision context. With these points in mind, there are several core tenets of SFT that can be integrated into most training activities. For example, Fiske (2007) described how trainers can model and incorporate the three pragmatic guidelines of SFT (if it's not broken, don't fix it; if it works, do more of it; if it doesn't work, do something different) into their training activities. This might involve encouraging trainees to identify and build on their clinical strengths while using these strengths to improve what is not working well for them or their clients. SFT trainers also encourage self-reflection, small-group work, and other experiential activities to help trainees come to their own conclusions about the usefulness and possibilities of SFT in their work. See Fiske (2007) for more ideas about implementing a solution-focused approach to SFT training.

Supervision offers similar opportunities to apply solution-focused thinking and techniques (Thomas, 2013). For example, solution-focused supervisors can establish supervisee-driven goals at the start of supervision. They can also request ongoing feedback from supervisees on their progress toward goals and the usefulness of supervision for them. Supervisors can explore and build on the supervisee's progress, exceptions, and other resources relevant to their desired outcomes from supervision. As time goes on, trainers will develop additional ways to incorporate solution-focused principles and practices into SFT supervision, workshops, consultations, and other training activities.

Use Crib Sheets at First

Learning SFT is a daunting task that requires patience and persistence on the part of trainers and trainees. Although SFT is conceptually simpler than other approaches, the skills required to properly implement it can be very challenging at first. These skills include building a repertoire of useful questions, formulating "next questions" based on clients' exact words, and staying with one major SFT task instead of moving back and forth between tasks. One way to expedite the learning process is to use simple outlines or *crib sheets* that include major tasks and questions addressed in SFT sessions. Appendix B provides crib sheets for first and later sessions in SFT. Although crib sheets are more useful in the early stages of learning, experienced therapists may also benefit from periodically reviewing and using them in their work.

Use Experiential Training Formats

Comedian–musician Martin Mull reportedly observed that "writing about music is like dancing about architecture." The same holds true for therapy training in that writing, reading, or talking about an approach is insufficient in helping people apply it with proficiency. Gaining knowledge of SFT principles and practices through readings and other sources is a good starting point. However, when it comes to developing proficiency in the approach, there is no substitute for *practicing* and *doing*. The four-step "say/show/practice/feedback" process offers great promise for training and supervision in SFT.

1. **Say (describe the approach or skill being taught).** When possible, provide trainees with basic readings, handouts, slides, or other information prior to the training session. In the session itself, it may be helpful to briefly review basic SFT information and terminology in conjunction with the visual and hands-on activities described below.
2. **Show (use videos and real-time demonstrations).** Videos and onsite demonstrations bring SFT to life for trainees who may have little or no experience with the approach. Real-time demonstrations provide

a shared experience that can be revisited throughout the training day to clarify SFT principles and practices. Another benefit of videos and demonstrations is that trainers can stop at various points in the conversation to ask trainees what they would ask next, follow up on or let go, or come back to later—along with the rationale for their choices. If training occurs over several weeks or months, as it does in supervision, demonstrations can be revisited as often as needed to optimize their impact.

3. **Practice (allow sufficient time to practice skills).** The skill-building benefits of short, structured, deliberate practice sessions have been verified in studies of high-performing athletes, musicians, and others (Ericsson & Pool, 2016). There is preliminary evidence that deliberate practice activities can improve the effectiveness of psychotherapists, particularly when those activities require the trainee or therapist to respond to simulations of difficult therapy situations (Chow et al., 2015). SFT trainers often encourage hands-on practice activities during and between training sessions. These activities may range from 5-minute workshop exercises to whole-session videotapes that trainees submit for coaching and feedback from the trainer. In addition to practicing specific SFT techniques, trainees should be encouraged to practice other "facilitative interpersonal skills" (T. Anderson et al., 2020) linked to common factors and effective outcomes. These skills include therapist empathy, warmth, hopefulness, responsiveness, and other skills that enhance outcomes regardless of one's therapy approach.

4. **Feedback (provide frequent and targeted feedback).** Targeted feedback is detailed, specific to the skill being taught, and linked to the goals of trainees and training. This type of feedback is more feasible in ongoing supervision relationships or intensive training programs than it is in single day workshops. If trainers cannot meet individually with trainees for several sessions (which is often the case), they can model targeted feedback in response to videos and demonstrations used during training; for example, the trainer can show a portion of videotape and point out specific therapist techniques, errors, and other relevant aspects of the client–therapist exchange. Trainees can

also be encouraged to seek out targeted feedback from their colleagues and supervisors, and to provide such feedback to themselves as a form of self-supervision.

Address Common Obstacles, Misconceptions, and Questions

Several commonly encountered obstacles, misunderstandings, and questions may arise as practitioners begin learning about and implementing SFT.

Common Obstacles

When possible, it is useful to focus a portion of training on each of the following areas.

Slowing Down and Staying With. One of the most difficult skills for people new to SFT is slowing down and staying with clients and topics long enough to elicit useful details and descriptions. Trainees are often surprised when they initially observe the patient, slow-paced conversations that occur between clients and experienced solution-focused therapists. As Shennan (2019) noted, "a typical solution-focused session is peppered with pauses, while either the worker is considering their next question or the client is thinking of an answer. A slow pace is useful for solution-focused work" (p. 196).

Constructing Next Questions. Although crib sheets help therapists initiate a solution-focused question, they cannot help them ask effective follow-up or "next" questions. This is because next questions are constructed on the fly from the client's previous response and exact words. When possible, SFT trainings should include exercises in which trainees practice listening to the client's responses and constructing next questions.

Shifting From Problem-Focused to Solution-Focused Practice. The process of becoming solution-focused often requires a significant perceptual and behavioral shift from problem-focused ideas and techniques. It is useful to prepare trainees for this process by encouraging them to be patient with themselves (and their colleagues and agencies), to regularly remind themselves why they want to practice SFT, to connect with SFT practitioners and online discussion groups, and to find ways to enjoy the learning process as much as possible.

Common Misconceptions

As discussed in Chapter 5, SFT has been mistakenly characterized as ignoring client problems and emotions, being mechanistic or solution-forced, and being ineffective with clients who experience traumas and other serious problems. These misconceptions should be proactively addressed in university training programs, workshops, and other training contexts to promote a more accurate understanding of SFT and its evidence base.

Common Questions

Although each training group is unique and will have its own questions, it is helpful to be prepared for questions that regularly come up in SFT trainings such as the ones below (Murphy, 2023).

Do Clients Ever Get Frustrated by All the Questions? Sometimes they do, but most clients will answer them because they realize the therapist is "on their side" and the questions are directly linked to their desired outcomes. Solution-focused therapists ask hard questions that require hard work from clients. Although it would be easier on clients if the therapist would assess the problem and tell them what to do about it, that is not the solution-focused way. Most clients realize that early in the process and appreciate the opportunity to develop their own solutions.

How Does SFT Address Multicultural Issues? SFT has flourished in many cultures and countries and includes several features of culturally responsive services (De Jong & Berg, 2013; Neipp & Beyebach, 2022). SFT tenets and techniques are also supported by the diversity-based values, ethical codes, and practice standards of professional organizations and licensing boards governing the practice of psychology, counseling, social work, and allied professions. Chapter 3 provides a more detailed discussion of SFT's multicultural orientation and effectiveness.

Does SFT Work for Serious Problems? Although this question was addressed in Chapter 5, it is included here because it frequently comes up in SFT trainings. As a reminder, research findings support SFT's overall effectiveness with trauma survivors and other clients who experience problems labeled as serious, deep-seated, and significant. For example, a recent examination of six well-designed outcome studies provided evidence that SFT was effective with clients dealing with various traumas (Eads & Lee, 2019). When responding to this question in training situations, trainers can cite the above findings and refer people to Froerer et al. (2018) for more information on the use of SFT with clients experiencing traumas such as physical and sexual abuse, domestic violence, sex trafficking, and posttraumatic stress disorder.

Evaluate the Usefulness and Impact of Training

This suggestion encourages trainers to evaluate SFT trainings with attention to their usefulness and impact for trainees and their clients. Evaluating training sessions and programs might include gathering information on pre- and posttraining differences in trainees' (a) knowledge of SFT principles and practices, including key distinctions between solution-focused and problem-focused approaches; (b) everyday clinical practices; (c) client outcomes; and (d) other factors related to the goals of training and trainees.

SUMMARY

Chapter 6 has offered suggestions for future developments in SFT research, practice, and training. Research suggestions included increasing the number of well-designed outcome studies, meta-analyses, and micro-analyses of SFT in as many different countries and cultures as possible; encouraging practitioners to collect practice-based evidence using feedback measures and other forms of client input; and examining the impact of cultural factors on therapy outcomes. Suggestions for future practice included adopting a multicultural orientation and scientist–practitioner approach to clinical work; connecting with solution-focused colleagues, organizations, and other resources; using teletherapy and other technology applications to expand the impact and reach of SFT; and maintaining a sense of wonder, curiosity, and appreciation. Training suggestions included walking the walk by adopting solution-focused methods of training, using experiential training formats, and evaluating the impact and benefit of training for trainees and their clients. It is safe to say that the future of solution-focused research, practice, and training is full of possibilities, and that future developments in these areas will be driven by the pragmatic question that has guided SFT for several decades: *What do therapists and clients talk about when therapy is effective?*

7

Summary

From its humble beginnings in Milwaukee, solution-focused therapy (SFT) has become one of the most popular and fastest-growing approaches in the world because it is evidence based, efficient, and culturally responsive. SFT (also called solution-focused brief therapy or SFBT) is a collaborative approach that invites clients to describe what they want from therapy and to apply what they already have toward achieving it.

Led by de Shazer and Berg, the Milwaukee group spent countless hours in the evidence-based process of watching therapy sessions to identify and replicate what therapists and clients talked about when therapy was successful. Their discoveries led to an unconventional therapy approach that challenged longstanding precepts and practices of the psychotherapy profession.

- **Nothing happens all the time, including the client's problem.** This obvious observation led to the not-so-obvious strategy of building on

https://doi.org/10.1037/0000370-007
Solution-Focused Therapy, by J. J. Murphy

"exceptions" or solutions that were already happening, just not as often as preferred. Clients became more encouraged and hopeful when they realized they already had what they needed to move forward in their lives. Increasing the frequency and magnitude of exceptions is a hallmark of SFT that reflects the approach's emphasis on simplicity, minimalism, and pragmatism.

- **Client–therapist dialogue is a powerful mechanism of change.** As the team continued to gather evidence, they discovered that the coconstruction of solutions through client–therapist dialogue was the primary means of change in SFT—a discovery verified by microanalyses of the approach (Bavelas, 2012; Bavelas et al., 2014; Korman et al., 2013). The postmodern, social constructionist notion of cocreating solutions through client–therapist dialogue challenged modernist ideas about how and why psychotherapy worked.

- **The more collaborative the therapy, the better the outcomes.** SFT is a radically collaborative, client-directed approach that centralizes and privileges the goals, resources, and input of clients throughout the therapy process. Clients are invited to participate in every aspect of their care to the extent that they are able and willing to do so. Research on multicultural counseling and common factors indicates that centralizing clients in these ways enhances the likelihood of providing effective, culturally responsive, socially just therapy services (Norcross & Lambert, 2019; D. W. Sue et al., 2019).

The evidence-based practices of the Milwaukee group have been sustained and adapted by subsequent generations of solution-focused therapists from every continent and applied with clients from a diverse range of cultures, racial/ethnic backgrounds, and intersectional identities.

SFT THEORY AND PROCESS

Chapters 3 and 4 provided detailed descriptions and illustrations of SFT theory and process in action. The following discussion summarizes these core components of the approach.

Theory

SFT theory was developed by analyzing effective client–therapist inter-actions, repeating what worked and discarding what didn't, and continually refining the approach in response to new evidence. In contrast to the broad scope of other theories, SFT theory focuses on client–therapist interactions *within* the therapy context. The pragmatic focus of SFT theory and practice is reflected in three practical guidelines: If it's not broken, don't fix it; if it works, do more of it; if it doesn't work, do something differ-ent. SFT theory also includes the following tenets: clients are resourceful and cooperative, nothing happens constantly, small changes can lead to big changes, the solution is not necessarily related to the problem, and the language of solutions is different from the language of problems.

Process

The collaborative nature of SFT is evident in the cultural humility of the therapist, active involvement of the client, and key tasks and techniques of the approach.

Role of the Therapist, Client, and Client–Therapist Relationship

The role of the solution-focused therapist "tends to be more egalitarian and democratic" than the more authoritarian therapist role in other approaches (de Shazer et al., 2021, p. 3). Solution-focused therapists approach clients from a stance of cultural humility and not knowing. They accept clients' statements and perceptions at face value and refrain from "making any interpretations about the meanings behind their wants, needs, or behaviors" (de Shazer et al., 2021, p. 4). These attitudes and actions serve to centralize the client, decentralize the therapist, and foster the type of client engage-ment and collaboration associated with successful outcomes (Tryon et al., 2019). They also reflect egalitarian principles of multiculturalism and social justice.

The client-directed focus of SFT is reflected in the notion that *the therapist works for the client, not the other way around.* This does not mean the role of the client is easy. Solution-focused questions are hard to answer, and therapists typically stay with a question or topic for as long as it takes to elicit a clear response or description. The coconstruction of solutions requires persistence and patience from therapists and clients alike. This is one of the reasons SFT is considered "simple but not easy"—simple to understand but far from easy to do because it requires a large measure of therapist restraint, concentration, and trust in clients' capabilities.

The collaborative client–therapist relationship in SFT is evident in every phase of the work from establishing a therapy direction through deciding when to end services. Giving clients a central voice in their care strengthens the therapeutic alliance, improves outcomes, and enhances clients' investment in therapy and ownership of therapeutic gains and successes.

Tasks and Techniques

The following tasks represent the entirety of solution-focused practice and occur in varying degrees and sequences in most SFT sessions.

Task 1: Setting a Direction. SFT begins by eliciting clients' best hopes (desired outcome) from therapy and eliciting a detailed description of how their lives would be different should they achieve the outcome (preferred future or solution description). Therapists ask the miracle question, tomorrow question, or similar question—along with detail-gathering "What else?" questions—to elicit a detailed description of actions, thoughts, feelings, social relationships, and other positive differences that make up the client's preferred future. Recall from Chapter 4 that Jalen's desired outcome was "getting out into it and being more social." With the help of the tomorrow question and several "what else?" questions, Jalen was able to describe a multifaceted preferred future consisting of concrete differences he would notice as he became more social. Establishing a client-selected direction is the foundation for everything that follows in SFT.

Task 2: Building on Exceptions and Other Resources. Once a direction is established, therapists assist clients in building on exceptions (or instances of the preferred future) and other relevant inner and outer resources. When exceptions are discovered, therapists explore related details with emphasis on the client's contributions ("How did you make it happen?"). Jalen was able identify several exceptions to his self-described "antisocial problem" (e.g., phone call, trip to the grocery store) and other resources that could assist him in becoming more social (e.g., church friends, sense of humor). The practicality and efficiency of constructing solutions from naturally occurring aspects of clients' lives has made this task a hallmark of SFT throughout its history.

Task 3: Exploring Progress. The main purpose of exploring client progress in SFT is to facilitate change-focused conversations related to desired outcomes. For example, requesting the client's 0–10 rating of where they are in relation to their preferred future creates several solution-building options ("Why isn't it lower?" "How did you move up a full point from last time?" "How have you kept things from getting worse?"). SFT therapists explore progress using informal scaling questions ("On a scale of 0 to 10 . . .") or formal scales like the Outcome Rating Scale (ORS). Jalen's total ORS scores across sessions were 21.6, 18.9, 28.2, and 29.3. The therapist kept the ORS in plain sight during therapy sessions, occasionally referring to Jalen's ratings to offer a comment or question ("Your ratings in every area are higher than they were 3 weeks ago, and your total score is over 9 points higher. How would you explain that?"). As seen with Jalen and others, exploring and empowering progress encourages clients to reflect on and own their hard-won gains and victories.

The *three main techniques* or activities of SFT are *asking* useful questions, *listening* attentively to clients' answers, and *amplifying* aspects of clients and their lives that support desired outcomes. When being purely solution-focused, there is rarely anything the therapist does outside of these activities.

EVALUATION AND EVIDENCE BASE

Evaluation and evidence-based practice have played prominent roles in the development and evolution of SFT. The approach itself was constructed from observational evidence of what clients and therapists talked about when therapy was effective. As noted in Chapter 5, the empirical support for the processes and effectiveness of SFT has come from *outcome research* (randomized controlled trials, meta-analyses, and other research reviews);

process research (microanalyses of SFT processes and mechanisms of change); and *common factors research* (empirical findings on nonspecific ingredients of effective therapy).

The combination of over 150 randomized controlled trials, numerous meta-analyses and research reviews, and other outcome studies indicate that SFT is a transculturally effective approach with a diverse range of clients, difficulties, and contexts including: adults and children from all parts of the world; internalizing and externalizing problems, traumas, relationship problems, domestic violence, substance misuse, schizophrenia, and self-harming; and service contexts and settings such as coaching, community planning, schools, hospitals, clinics, businesses, correctional facilities, crisis hotlines, law enforcement agencies, and more. SFT yields effect sizes equal to those of cognitive behavior therapy and other evidence-based approaches, and often does so in fewer average sessions (Gingerich et al., 2012; Kim et al., 2019).

The efficiency of SFT is particularly appealing to clients who cannot commit to long-term therapy for logistical or financial reasons. The client-directed, strengths-based focus of SFT is less invasive than the more authoritarian, interpretive, therapist-driven style of other approaches. These features help to explain why SFT is considered a culturally responsive and socially just approach (Kim, 2014; Murphy & Sparks, 2018)—and why it is considered "an excellent first-choice evidence-based psychotherapy for most psychological, behavioral, and relational problems" (Dolan & Trepper, 2021, p. xviii).

When choosing from among the growing number of evidence-based psychotherapies, students and practitioners can replace the outdated question "Which therapy approach is the best?" with "What therapy approach do I want to use with my clients?" Given that all evidence-based approaches seem to work equally well, each therapist can confidently choose an approach that reflects how they want to relate to clients and who they want to be as a therapist. This book provided many reasons why more and more therapists are using SFT to help their clients change with dignity.

Appendix A: Commonly Used Questions in Solution-Focused Therapy

The following questions can be used to address the tasks of setting a direction, building on exceptions and other resources, and exploring progress in SFT.

Setting a Direction

Desired Outcome

- What are your best hopes from this meeting?
- How will you know it was useful?
- What will be different for you if this ends up helping?
- How will you know it was worthwhile to come here today?

Preferred Future

- (*Miracle question—condensed version*) If a miracle happened while you were sleeping tonight and this problem vanished, what is the first thing you would notice tomorrow morning to tell you the miracle happened? Then what? What else?

- (*Tomorrow question*) If you woke up tomorrow having achieved your hope of [insert client's desired outcome], what would you notice first? Next? What else?
- What would be the first small sign that [insert client's desired outcome]? What else?
- Who else will notice? How might they respond? What would that be like for you?

Building on Exceptions and Other Resources

Exceptions

- Has anything been better since you scheduled this appointment?
- What small pieces of the miracle/tomorrow day you just described have happened recently?
- Of all the things you described, which ones are happening even just a little?
- What puts you at 3 and not 0? What's different about 3 than 0? How did you get from a lower number to 3?
- What do you want to continue happening in your life?
- Tell me about a tiny bright spot in your week. How did you make it happen? What does that say about you? What has it taught you about yourself?
- Who else noticed? How did they react? What was that like for you?
- What will it take to make it happen more often?

Other Resources

- How have you handled other challenges? How might that help you now?
- Of everything you've tried so far, what has been most helpful?
- What have you thought about doing but haven't tried yet?
- Who helps you the most when you have a problem? What do they do that is helpful? How might you use that (or their help) now?
- How did you do learn to knit/roller blade/play piano/. . .? How could that help you now?
- How do you manage to keep going?

- Who do you respect most? What advice would they offer?
- What advice might you give others in this situation?

Exploring Progress

- What's better since our last meeting?
- On a scale of 0 to 10, where 10 is [client's desired outcome] and 0 is the exact opposite, where would you put yourself now? Has it ever been lower? [If client says "yes"] What's different now compared to then? How did you move to a higher number?

When Clients Report Improvements

- How did you go from a 3 to a 4? [referring to client's higher Outcome Rating Scale or 0–10 rating]
- What are you doing differently now? How did you think of doing that?
- What do these changes say about you? What have you learned about yourself?
- Who else noticed? How did they respond? What was that like for you?
- What advice would you offer someone who wants to make similar changes?
- What would your partner/friends/kids/parents be noticing if you were a half point higher? What else would they notice?
- What will be the first small sign that things are getting a little better? What might help make that happen?

When Clients Report No Change or Decline

- With all you've been through, how have you managed to keep going?
- How have you kept things from getting worse?
- What helps you stay at it and keep trying?
- What has kept you from giving up?
- How could you keep the number from dropping further?
- What would your partner/friends/kids/parents be noticing if you were a half point higher? What else would they notice?
- What will be the first small sign that things are holding steady or getting a little better? What might help make that happen?

Appendix B:
SFT Crib Sheets for
First and Later Sessions

The following crib sheets can be used to guide first and later sessions in solution-focused therapy (SFT). They should be applied in a flexible manner and adapted to the client and situation. Some items, such as the Outcome Rating Scale (ORS) and Session Rating Scale (SRS), are listed as optional because they are not a standard part of SFT.

Adapted from *Solution-Focused Counseling in Schools* (4th ed., pp. 382–383), by J. J. Murphy, 2023, American Counseling Association. Copyright 2023 by American Counseling Association. Adapted with permission.

SFT Crib Sheet (First Session)

Client's Name: _____ Session Number: _____ Date: _____

Opening (Optional)

Interests, talents, skills?

Desired Outcome

Best hopes from therapy? How will you know this was useful?

Optional—Use/discuss ORS

Preferred Future

Miracle/tomorrow question

What would you notice first? What else? What else?

Miracle/tomorrow scale

Where would you put yourself now (0–10)? _____

Good enough number to end therapy (0–10)? _____

Optional—Use confidence/willingness scales:

Confidence in achieving desired outcome/goal (0–10)? _____

Willingness to work toward it (0–10)? _____

Exceptions (and Other Resources)

When doesn't the problem happen? Pieces or instances of preferred future already happening?

Details/differences: When? Where? How? What was different? Who noticed? How did you make it happen?

Other inner/outer resources: Who/what else might help? How do you keep going?

Closing

Acknowledge client's struggles, hopes, exceptions, inner/outer resources.

Ask about next signs/next steps toward desired outcome.

Suggest observation or action experiment.

Discuss termination if client nears good enough number.

Optional—Use/discuss SRS

SFT Crib Sheet (Later Session)

Client's Name: _____ Session Number: _____ Date: _____

Explore Progress

What's better since previous session? Where are you on miracle/tomorrow scale (0–10)?

Optional—Use/discuss ORS

If Things are Better

Explore details: How did you do it? What's different as a result? Who else noticed?

If Things are Same or Worse

Explore coping/resilience: How do you keep going? How have you kept things from getting worse?

Revisit Desired Outcome (as needed)

Is it still important? Achievable?

Exceptions (and Other Resources)

Explore exceptions and other resources discovered in this or prior sessions.

Closing

Acknowledge client's struggles, hopes, exceptions, inner/outer resources.

Ask about next signs/next steps toward desired outcome.

Suggest observation or action experiment.

Discuss termination if client nears good enough number.

Optional—Use/discuss SRS.

Appendix C:
Client Feedback Scales From Partners for Change Outcome Management System (PCOMS)

The Outcome Rating Scale (ORS) and Session Rating Scale (SRS) are part of the evidence-based Partners for Change Outcome Management System (PCOMS; Duncan & Sparks, 2018). Each four-item scale can be administered and scored in about 1 minute using a paper-and-pencil format or a laptop, smartphone, tablet, or other digital device. Clients indicate their perceptions by placing a mark on each of the four lines or using their finger on a digital device. Scoring is done by hand or digitally using a web-based system such as Better Outcomes Now (Duncan, 2023; https:// www.betteroutcomesnow.com). Web-based applications automatically calculate and graph client ratings across sessions.

The ORS is administered at the start of (or just before) each session to obtain clients' ratings of how they are doing in the following domains: Individually (personal well-being), Interpersonally (family, intimate relationships), Socially (work, school, peers), and Overall. Clients mark each 10-centimeter line (domain), and the total score is the sum of all four domains to the nearest millimeter. Clients complete the SRS at the end of each session to indicate their experience of the following areas of the client–therapist alliance: Relationship (feeling heard and respected),

Goals and Topics (importance of topics discussed), Approach or Method (goodness of fit between therapist's approach and client), and Overall (overall effectiveness of the session). The total score is the sum of all four areas to the nearest millimeter (0–34 = weak alliance, 35–38 = fair alliance, 39–40 = strong alliance). The main purpose and benefit of the SRS is to detect and correct emerging alliance problems. Lower SRS scores are welcomed and discussed in a candid, nondefensive way (Murphy & Duncan, 2007). PCOMS includes child versions of both scales for use with children 12 and under, and group versions of the SRS and child SRS.

There is growing evidence that using PCOMS to collect formal, systematic client feedback improves therapy outcomes regardless of one's therapy approach (Lambert et al., 2019). Client feedback enables practitioners to monitor the client's response to therapy and adjust services accordingly. Although informal scales have been used in solution-focused therapy (SFT) for decades, formal scaling is not considered a standard part of solution-focused work. However, several writers have urged their solution-focused colleagues to consider incorporating PCOMS into their practice because it is supported by research and consistent with SFT's client-centered emphasis (De Jong & Berg, 2013; Gillaspy & Murphy, 2012; Ratner & Yusuf, 2015; Trepper & Franklin, 2012). After all, "experimenting with new practices that enhance 'what works' in therapy is in the spirit of discovery that led to the original development of solution-focused practice" (De Jong & Berg, 2013, p. 254).

The relative impact of using PCOMS or other evidence-based feedback systems in SFT, compared with using only informal scales or both, is an empirical question that warrants additional investigation. Refer to Duncan and Sparks (2018) for detailed information on the development, rationale, and implementation of PCOMS, and to https://www.betteroutcomesnow. com for additional articles, writings, videos, and other PCOMS-related resources.

APPENDIX C

Outcome Rating Scale (ORS)

Name _____ Age (Yrs): ____ Gender: _____

Session # ____ Date: _____

Who is filling out this form? Please check one: Self _____ Other _____

If other, what is your relationship to this person? _____

Looking back over the last week, including today, help us understand how you have been feeling by rating how well you have been doing in the following areas of your life, where marks to the left represent low levels and marks to the right indicate high levels. *If you are filling out this form for another person, please fill out according to how you think he or she is doing.*

Individually

(Personal well-being)

I————————————————I

Interpersonally

(Family, close relationships)

I————————————————I

Socially

(Work, school, friendships)

I————————————————I

Overall

(General sense of well-being)

I————————————————I

Session Rating Scale (SRS V.3.0)

Name _____ Age (Yrs): ____ Gender: _____

Session # ____ Date: _____

Please rate today's session by placing a mark on the line nearest to the description that best fits your experience.

Relationship

| I did not feel heard, understood, and respected. | I——————————————————I | I felt heard, understood, and respected. |

Goals and Topics

| We did not work on or talk about what I wanted to work on and talk about. | I——————————————————I | We worked on or talked about what I wanted to work on and talk about. |

Approach or Method

| The therapist's approach is not a good fit for me. | I——————————————————I | The therapist's approach is a good fit for me. |

Overall

| There was something missing in the session today. | I——————————————————I | Overall, today's session was right for me. |

Note. Copyright 2002 by S. D. Miller, B. L. Duncan, and L. D. Johnson. Permission to publish the PCOMS family of instruments granted by Barry L. Duncan. Depicted measures are for examination only. Download free working copy in 35 languages at https://www.betteroutcomesnow.com/.

Glossary of Key Terms

AMPLIFYING   Highlighting, detailing, and expanding on aspects of clients' lives that support their desired outcomes; examples include asking "What else?" and other detail-gathering questions, making lists, acknowledging, complimenting, validating, echoing, and summarizing; one of the three main techniques of solution-focused therapy.

ASKING   Constructing questions that elicit, explore, and expand on what clients want from therapy, what they already have toward achieving it, and progress toward achieving it; one of the three main techniques of solution-focused therapy.

BUILDING ON EXCEPTIONS   Three-step method of eliciting, exploring, and expanding the presence and impact of exceptions in the lives of clients; also called 3-E PROCESS OF BUILDING ON EXCEPTIONS; part of the second main task of solution-focused therapy (building on exceptions and other resources).

BUILDING ON OTHER RESOURCES   Three-step method of eliciting, exploring, and expanding the impact of inner/outer resources in the lives of clients; also called 3-E PROCESS OF BUILDING ON RESOURCES;

part of the second main task of solution-focused therapy (building on exceptions and other resources).

CULTURAL HUMILITY   A stance of respectful openness toward clients in which the therapist approaches every client as a culture of one and every conversation as a cross-cultural exchange; central feature of a multicultural orientation.

DESIRED OUTCOME   General statement of what the client wants from therapy; first component of setting a direction for therapy; also called HOPED-FOR OUTCOME, DESTINATION, ENDPOINT, or GOAL.

EXCEPTIONS   Situations or times in which the problem is absent or less noticeable; pieces or instances of the client's preferred future that have happened or are happening, just not as often as desired.

EXPLORING PROGRESS   Measuring and responding to client reports of progress in ways that facilitate desired outcomes; one of the three main tasks of solution-focused therapy.

LISTENING   Attending to clients' exact words with a constructive ear tuned to hints of hope, strength, success, and other aspects of clients and their lives that support desired outcomes; one of the three main techniques of solution-focused therapy.

MICROANALYSIS   Method of process research that closely examines the sequence and content of client–therapist interactions to better understand how communication works in therapy; used to examine the coconstructive process of solution-focused therapy.

MIRACLE QUESTION   Classic solution-focused method of eliciting and exploring the client's preferred future by obtaining a detailed description of life without the problem: "Suppose that a miracle happened tonight, while you were asleep, and this problem was solved. How would you know? What would be different?"

OUTCOME RATING SCALE (ORS)   Ultra-brief, four-item rating scale used to obtain session-by-session client feedback on progress toward desired outcomes; part of Partners for Change Outcome Management System (PCOMS); see Appendix C.

PARTNERS FOR CHANGE OUTCOME MANAGEMENT SYSTEM (PCOMS)   Evidence-based system of obtaining session-by-session client feedback of progress toward desired outcomes and therapeutic alliance using the Outcome Rating Scale (ORS) and Session Rating Scale (SRS), respectively; see Appendix C for more information.

PREFERRED FUTURE   Detailed, multifaceted description of clients' desired outcome that includes specific differences they would notice in themselves, key relationships, and other aspects of life should they achieve the outcome; second component of setting a direction for therapy; also called SOLUTION DESCRIPTION or MIRACLE DESCRIPTION.

PRETREATMENT (OR PRESESSION) CHANGE   Desired change that occurs between the client's decision to seek formal assistance and the first therapy session.

SCALING   Formal or informal questions/methods that invite clients to rate their position, progress, or other factors on a 0–10 (or similar) scale; versatile technique that serves many purposes in solution-focused therapy.

SESSION RATING SCALE   Ultra-brief, four-item rating scale used to obtain session-by-session client feedback on the therapeutic alliance; part of Partners for Change Outcome Management System (PCOMS); see Appendix C.

SETTING A DIRECTION   Identifying what clients want from therapy (desired outcome) and how their lives would be different should they achieve it (preferred future); the first main task of solution-focused therapy.

SOCIAL CONSTRUCTIONISM   Postmodern theory that depicts therapy as a coconstructive process in which new meanings are coconstructed through client–therapist dialogue.

SOLUTION-FOCUSED THERAPY (SFT)   A collaborative approach that invites clients to describe what they want from therapy and apply what they already have toward achieving it in the shortest time possible.

SOLUTION TALK   Questions, comments, and conversations about clients' desired outcomes, preferred futures, exceptions, resources, and progress toward desired outcomes.

TOMORROW QUESTION   Used in place of the miracle question to elicit the client's preferred future: "If you woke up tomorrow having achieved your hope of (client's desired outcome), what is the first thing you would notice?"

Suggested Readings and Resources

The number of reading materials, professional organizations, videos, podcasts, discussion groups, and other solution-focused therapy (SFT) resources has increased steadily over the years. The following represent a few of these resources.

INTERNATIONAL SFT DISCUSSION GROUP

In 1995, Harry Korman started an online SFT discussion group (https://www.sikt.nu/sft-l) for raising questions, sharing ideas and resources, and participating in a worldwide community of people interested in solution-focused practice. The list has grown steadily and remains a major means of international communication about SFT.

PROFESSIONAL ASSOCIATIONS

The following associations are a few of the many solution-focused professional organizations around the world. The best way to find out if there is a solution-focused association in your area is to post a note on the international SFT discussion group described above (https://www.sikt.nu/sft-l).

Australasian Solution Focused Association (**ASFA**; https://www.solutionfocused.org.au)

Formed in 2013, the ASFA promotes the use of solution-focused practice in therapy and other contexts in Australia and New Zealand. The ASFA hosts an annual conference and ongoing training courses on SFT.

European Brief Therapy Association (EBTA; https://www.ebta.eu)
EBTA offers regular conferences, the SFT evaluation/research list, and other solution-focused resources and information.

Solution-Focused Brief Therapy Association (SFBTA; https://www.sfbta.org)
Based in America, SFBTA hosts an annual conference and offers a running list of SFT research studies as well as books, training videos, SFT archives, and links to other websites.

Solution-Focused Institute of South Africa (https://www.solutionfocusedsa.com)
The Institute is run by Jacqui von Cziffra-Bergs and offers online and in-person training workshops and courses, books, and videos on solution-focused practice.

TRAINING RESOURCES

Books

Nelson, T. S. (Ed.). (2014). *Education and training in solution-focused brief therapy.* Haworth Press.

Rohrig, P., & Clarke, J. (Eds.). (2008). *57 solution-focused activities for facilitators and consultants.* Solutions Books.

Videos/DVDs

Psychotherapy.net, Victor Yalom's company, offers training videos on various psychotherapies, including SFT. Several videos feature interviews and therapy sessions with SFT cofounder Insoo Berg Kim as well as other solution-focused therapists.

Alexander Street (https://www.alexanderstreet.com) is an online audio/video streaming service that offers videos on SFT and other psychotherapy and counseling approaches.

Podcasts

The following websites feature interviews with SFT practitioners and authors on topics related to solution-focused practice, research, and training:

https://www.sfontour.com/simplyfocuspodcast (produced by Elfie Czerny and Dominik Godat)

https://sfpodcast.podbean.com/ (produced by UK Association for Solution Focused Practice)

www.hbtc.ca/podcast (produced by Halifax Brief Therapy Centre)

RESEARCH LISTS

Lists of SFT research studies can be found on websites of the Solution-Focused Brief Therapy Association (https://www.sfbta.org) and European Brief Therapy Association (https://www.ebta.eu).

RECOMMENDED READINGS

Between 1982 and 1995, de Shazer published five books that capture SFT's shift from studying therapist interventions ("What do therapists say and do when therapy is effective?") to examining the coconstructive impact of therapist–client dialogue ("What do therapists and clients talk about when therapy is effective?"). If you can read only a few of his works, I would recommend *Keys to Solution in Brief Therapy* (de Shazer, 1985), *Words Were Originally Magic* (de Shazer, 1994), and *More Than Miracles* (de Shazer et al., 2021). *More Than Miracles*, de Shazer's last book, was originally published in 2007 and reissued with an updated preface in 2021. All three of these books are included in the following list of recommend readings.

Bavelas, J. B. (2012). Connecting the lab to the therapy room: Microanalysis, co-construction, and solution-focused brief therapy. In C. Franklin, T. Trepper, W. J. Gingerich, & E. McCollum (Eds.), *Solution-focused brief therapy: A handbook of evidence-based practice* (pp. 144–162). Oxford University Press.

De Jong, P., & Berg, I. K. (2013). *Interviewing for solutions* (4th ed.). Brooks/Cole.

de Shazer, S. (1985). *Keys to solution in brief therapy.* Norton.

de Shazer, S. (1994). *Words were originally magic.* Norton.

de Shazer, S., Dolan, Y., Korman, H., Trepper, T., McCollum, E., & Berg, I. K. (2021). *More than miracles: The state of the art of solution-focused brief therapy* (Classic edition). Routledge.

Duncan, B. L. (2014). *On becoming a better therapist: Evidence-based practice one client at a time* (2nd ed.). American Psychological Association.

Franklin, C., Trepper, T. S., Gingerich, W. J., & McCollum, E. E. (Eds.). (2012). *Solution-focused brief therapy: A handbook of evidence-based practice.* Oxford University Press.

Froerer, A. S., Von Cziffra-Bergs, J., Kim, J. S., & Connie, E. E. (Eds.). (2018). *Solution-focused brief therapy with clients managing trauma.* Oxford University Press.

Gillaspy, J. A., & Murphy, J. J. (2012). Incorporating outcome and session rating scales in solution-focused brief therapy. In C. Franklin, T. S. Trepper, W. J. Gingerich, & E. E. McCollum (Eds.), *Solution-focused brief therapy: A handbook of evidence-based practice* (pp. 73–93). Oxford University Press.

Kim, J. S. (Ed.). (2014). *Solution-focused brief therapy: A multicultural approach.* Sage.

Korman, H., De Jong, P., & Smock Jordan, S. (2020). Steve de Shazer's theory development. *Journal of Solution Focused Practices, 4*(2), 47–70. https://digitalscholarship.unlv.edu/journalsfp/vol4/iss2/5

Kort, B., Froerer, A., & Walker, C. (2021). Creating a common language: How solution-focused brief therapy reflects current principles of change and common factors. *Journal of Solution-Focused Practices, 5*(1), 1–41. https://digitalscholarship.unlv.edu/journalsfp/vol5/iss1/5

McKergow, M. (2021). *The next generation of solution focused practice: Stretching the world for new opportunities and progress.* Routledge.

Murphy, J. J. (2023). *Solution-focused counseling in schools* (4th ed.). American Counseling Association.

Norcross, J. C., & Lambert, M. J. (2019). Evidence-based psychotherapy relationship: The third task force. In J. C. Norcross & M. J. Lambert (Eds.), *Psychotherapy relationships that work: Vol. 1. Evidence-based therapist contributions* (3rd ed., pp. 1–23). Oxford University Press. https://doi.org/10.1093/med-psych/9780190843953.003.0001

Pichot, T., & Smock, S. A. (2009). *Solution-focused substance abuse treatment.* Routledge.

Ratner, H., George, E., & Iveson, C. (2012). *Solution-focused brief therapy: 100 key points and techniques.* Routledge.

Shennan, G. (2019). *Solution-focused practice: Effective communication to facilitate change* (2nd ed.). Red Globe Press.

References

American Psychological Association. (2017). *Multicultural guidelines: An ecological approach to context, identity, and intersectionality.* https://www.apa.org/about/policy/multicultural-guidelines.pdf

American Psychological Association Presidential Task Force on Evidence-Based Practice. (2006). Evidence-based practice in psychology. *American Psychologist, 61*(4), 271–285. https://doi.org/10.1037/0003-066X.61.4.271

Anderson, H. (2007). The heart and spirit of collaborative therapy: The philosophical stance—"A way of being" in relationship and conversation. In H. Anderson & D. Gehart (Eds.), *Collaborative therapy: Relationships and conversations that make a difference* (pp. 43–59). Routledge.

Anderson, H., & Goolishian, H. (1992). The client is the expert: A not-knowing approach to therapy. In S. McNamee & K. J. Gergen (Eds.), *Therapy as social construction* (pp. 25–39). Sage.

Anderson, T., Finkelstein, J. D., & Horvath, S. A. (2020). The facilitative interpersonal skills method: Difficult psychotherapy moments and appropriate therapist responsiveness. *Counselling & Psychotherapy Research, 22*(3), 463–469. https://doi.org/10.1002/capr.12302

Andrews, G., Basu, A., Cuijpers, P., Craske, M. G., McEvoy, P., English, C. L., & Newby, J. M. (2018). Computer therapy for the anxiety and depression disorders is effective, acceptable and practical health care: An updated meta-analysis. *Journal of Anxiety Disorders, 55*, 70–78. https://doi.org/10.1016/j.janxdis.2018.01.001

Bateson, G., Jackson, D. D., Haley, J., & Weakland, J. H. (1956). Toward a theory of schizophrenia. *Behavioral Science, 1*(4), 251–264. https://doi.org/10.1002/bs.3830010402

Bavelas, J. B. (2012). Connecting the lab to the therapy room: Microanalysis, co-construction, and solution-focused brief therapy. In C. Franklin,

T. Trepper, W. J. Gingerich, & E. E. McCollum (Eds.), *Solution-focused brief therapy: A handbook of evidence-based practice* (pp. 144–162). Oxford University Press. https://doi.org/10.1093/acprof:oso/9780195385724.003.0063

Bavelas, J. B., McGee, D., Phillips, B., & Routledge, R. (2000). Microanalysis of communication in psychotherapy. *Human Systems: The Journal of Systemic Consultation and Management, 11*(1), 47–66. https://web.uvic.ca/psyc/bavelas/2000microa.pdf

Bavelas, J. B., Smock Jordan, S., Korman, H., & De Jong, P. (2014). Is solution-focused brief therapy different? *Family Therapy Magazine, 13,* 19–23. https://web.uvic.ca/psyc/bavelas/2014%20AAMFT%20re%20SFBT.pdf

Berg, I. K., & de Shazer, S. (1993). Making numbers talk: Language in therapy. In S. Friedman (Ed.), *The new language of change: Constructive collaboration in psychotherapy* (pp. 5–24). Guilford Press.

Berg, I. K., & Dolan, Y. (2001). *Tales of solutions: A collection of hope-inspiring stories.* W. W. Norton.

Beyebach, M. (2014). Change factors in solution-focused brief therapy: A review of the Salamanca studies. *Journal of Systemic Therapies, 33*(1), 62–77. https://doi.org/10.1521/jsyt.2014.33.1.62

Beyebach, M., Neipp, M. C., Solanes-Puchol, Á., & Martín-Del-Río, B. (2021). Bibliometric differences between WEIRD and non-WEIRD countries in the outcome research on solution-focused brief therapy. *Frontiers in Psychology, 12,* 754885. https://doi.org/10.3389/fpsyg.2021.754885

Bohart, A. C., & Tallman, K. (2010). Clients: The neglected common factor in therapy. In B. L. Duncan, S. D. Miller, B. E. Wampold, & M. A. Hubble (Eds.), *The heart and soul of change: Delivering what works in therapy* (2nd ed., pp. 83–111). American Psychological Association. https://doi.org/10.1037/12075-003

Bordin, E. S. (1979). The generalizability of the psychoanalytic concept of the working alliance. *Psychotherapy: Theory, Research, & Practice, 16*(3), 252–260. https://doi.org/10.1037/h0085885

Boyd-Franklin, N., Cleek, E. N., Wofsy, M., & Mundy, B. (2013). *Therapy in the real world: Effective treatments for challenging problems.* Guilford Press.

Bronfenbrenner, U. (1979). *Ecology of human development: Experiments by nature and design.* Harvard University Press.

Cade, B. (2007). Springs, streams, and tributaries: A history of the brief, solution-focused approach. In T. S. Nelson & F. N. Thomas (Eds.), *Handbook of solution-focused brief therapy: Clinical applications* (pp. 25–64). Haworth Press.

California Evidence-Based Clearinghouse for Child Welfare. (2022). *Solution-based casework (SBC).* https://www.cebc4cw.org/program/solution-based-casework/

Cantwell, P., & Holmes, S. (1994). Social construction: A paradigm shift for systemic therapy and training. *Australian and New Zealand Journal of Family Therapy, 15*(1), 17–26. https://doi.org/10.1002/j.1467-8438.1994.tb00978.x

Castonguay, L. G., & Hill, C. E. (Eds.). (2017). *How and why are some therapists better than others?: Understanding therapist effects.* American Psychological Association. https://doi.org/10.1037/0000034-000

Chow, D. L., Miller, S. D., Seidel, J. A., Kane, R. T., Thornton, J. A., & Andrews, W. P. (2015). The role of deliberate practice in the development of highly effective psychotherapists. *Psychotherapy, 52*(3), 337–345. https://doi.org/10.1037/pst0000015

Corbin, J., & Strauss, A. (2015). *Basics of qualitative research: Techniques and procedures for developing grounded theory* (4th ed.). Sage.

Corey, G. (2023). *Theory and practice of group counseling* (10th ed.). Cengage.

Crethar, H. C., Torres Rivera, E., & Nash, S. (2008). In search of common threads: Linking multicultural, feminist, and social justice counseling paradigms. *Journal of Counseling and Development, 86*(3), 269–278. https://doi.org/10.1002/j.1556-6678.2008.tb00509.x

Davis, D. E., DeBlaere, C., Owen, J., Hook, J. N., Rivera, D. P., Choe, E., Van Tongeren, D. R., Worthington, E. L., & Placeres, V. (2018). The multicultural orientation framework: A narrative review. *Psychotherapy, 55*(1), 89–100. https://doi.org/10.1037/pst0000160

De Jong, P., Bavelas, J. B., & Korman, H. (2013). Introduction to using microanalysis to observe co-construction in psychotherapy. *Journal of Systemic Therapies, 32*(3), 17–30. https://doi.org/10.1521/jsyt.2013.32.3.17

De Jong, P., & Berg, I. K. (2013). *Interviewing for solutions* (4th ed.). Brooks/Cole.

De Jong, P., & Hopwood, L. E. (1996). Outcome research on treatment conducted at the Brief Family Therapy Center, 1992–1993. In S. D. Miller, M. A. Hubble, & B. L. Duncan (Eds.), *Handbook of solution-focused brief therapy* (pp. 272–298). Jossey-Bass.

De Jong, P., Jordan, S. S., Healing, S., & Gerwing, J. (2020). Building miracles in dialogue: Observing co-construction through a microanalysis of calibrating sequences. *Journal of Systemic Therapies, 39*(2), 84–108. https://doi.org/10.1521/jsyt.2020.39.2.84

de Shazer, S. (1982). *Patterns of brief therapy: An ecosystemic approach.* Guilford Press.

de Shazer, S. (1984). The death of resistance. *Family Process, 23*(1), 11–17. https://doi.org/10.1111/j.1545-5300.1984.00011.x

de Shazer, S. (1985). *Keys to solution in brief therapy.* W. W. Norton.

de Shazer, S. (1987). Minimal elegance. *The Family Therapy Networker, 11*(8), 57–60.

de Shazer, S. (1988). *Clues: Investigating solutions in brief therapy*. W. W. Norton.

de Shazer, S. (1991). *Putting difference to work*. W. W. Norton.

de Shazer, S. (1994). *Words were originally magic*. W. W. Norton.

de Shazer, S., Berg, I. K., Lipchik, E., Nunnally, E., Molnar, A., Gingerich, W., & Weiner-Davis, M. (1986). Brief therapy: Focused solution development. *Family Process, 25*(2), 207–221. https://doi.org/10.1111/j.1545-5300.1986.00207.x

de Shazer, S., Dolan, Y., Korman, H., Trepper, T., McCollum, E., & Berg, I. K. (2021). *More than miracles: The state of the art of solution-focused brief therapy*. Routledge.

Dolan, Y., & Trepper, T. (2021). Preface. In S. de Shazer, Y. Dolan, H. Korman, T. Trepper, E. McCollum, & I. K. Berg, *More than miracles: The state of the art of solution-focused brief therapy* (pp. xv–xxii). Routledge.

Dolan, Y. M. (1991). *Resolving sexual abuse. Solution-focused therapy and Ericksonian hypnosis for adult survivors*. W. W. Norton.

Dolan, Y. M. (2000). *One small step: Moving beyond trauma and therapy to a life of joy*. iUniverse.

Duncan, B. L. (2014). *On becoming a better therapist: Evidence-based practice one client at a time* (2nd ed.). American Psychological Association.

Duncan, B. L. (2023). Better Outcomes Now. https://betteroutcomesnow.com/#/

Duncan, B. L., & Sparks, J. A. (2018). *The Partners for Change Outcome Management System: An integrated e-learning manual for everything PCOMS*. Better Outcomes Now. https://betteroutcomesnow.com/products/downloadable-book/

Dweck, C. S. (2016). *Mindset: The new psychology of success* (Updated edition). Penguin Random House.

Dweck, C. S., & Master, A. (2008). Self-theories motivate self-regulated learning. In D. H. Schunk & B. J. Zimmerman (Eds.), *Motivation and self-regulated learning: Theory, research, and applications* (pp. 31–52). Lawrence Erlbaum.

Eads, R., & Lee, M. Y. (2019). Solution focused therapy for trauma survivors: A review of the outcome literature. *Journal of Solution-Focused Practices, 3*(1), 1–10. https://digitalscholarship.unlv.edu/journalsfp/vol3/iss1/9

Elkin, I., Shea, M. T., Watkins, J. T., Imber, S. D., Sotsky, S. M., Collins, J. F., Glass, D. R., Pilkonis, P. A., Leber, W. R., Docherty, J. P., Fiester, S. J., & Parloff, M. B. (1989). National Institute of Mental Health Treatment of Depression Collaborative Research Program: General effectiveness of treatments. *Archives of General Psychiatry, 46*(11), 971–982. https://doi.org/10.1001/archpsyc.1989.01810110013002

Elliott, R., Bohart, A. C., Watson, J. C., & Murphy, D. (2019). Empathy. In J. C. Norcross & M. J. Lambert (Eds.), *Psychotherapy relationships that work: Vol. 1. Evidence-based therapist contributions* (3rd ed., pp. 245–287). Oxford University Press. https://doi.org/10.1093/med-psych/9780190843953.003.0007

Enck, P., & Zipfel, S. (2019). Placebo effects in psychotherapy: A framework. *Frontiers in Psychiatry, 10,* 456. https://doi.org/10.3389/fpsyt.2019.00456

Ericsson, A., & Pool, R. (2016). *Peak: Secrets from the new science of expertise.* Houghton Mifflin.

Finsrud, I., Nissen-Lie, H. A., Vrabel, K., Høstmælingen, A., Wampold, B. E., & Ulvenes, P. G. (2022). It's the therapist and the treatment: The structure of common therapeutic relationship factors. *Psychotherapy Research, 32*(2), 139–150. https://doi.org/10.1080/10503307.2021.1916640

Fisch, R., Ray, W. A., & Schlanger, K. (2010). *Focused problem resolution: Selected papers of the MRI Brief Therapy Center.* Zeig, Tucker, & Theisen.

Fisch, R., Weakland, J. H., & Segal, L. (1982). *The tactics of change: Doing therapy briefly.* Jossey-Bass.

Fiske, H. (2007). Solution-focused training: The medium and the message. In T. S. Nelson & F. N. Thomas (Eds.), *Handbook of solution-focused brief therapy: Clinical applications* (pp. 317–342). Haworth Press.

Fiske, H. (2017). Solution-focused brief therapy and suicide prevention. *International Journal of Brief Therapy and Family Science, 7*(1), 1–2. https://doi.org/10.35783/ijbf.7.1_1

Flückiger, C., Del Re, A. C., Wampold, B. E., & Horvath, A. O. (2018). The alliance in adult psychotherapy: A meta-analytic synthesis. *Psychotherapy, 55*(4), 316–340. https://doi.org/10.1037/pst0000172

Frank, D. J., & Frank, J. B. (1991). *Persuasion and healing: A comparative study of psychotherapy* (3rd ed.). Johns Hopkins University Press. https://doi.org/10.56021/9780801840678

Franklin, C., Streeter, C. L., Webb, L., & Guz, S. (2018). *Solution-focused brief therapy in alternative schools: Ensuring student success and preventing dropout.* Routledge. https://doi.org/10.4324/9781315186245

Franklin, C., Zhang, A., Froerer, A., & Johnson, S. (2017). Solution-focused brief therapy: A systematic review and meta-summary of process research. *Journal of Marital and Family Therapy, 43*(1), 16–30. https://doi.org/10.1111/jmft.12193

Froerer, A. S., & Jordan, S. S. (2013). Identifying solution-building formulations through microanalysis. *Journal of Systemic Therapies, 32*(3), 60–73. https://doi.org/10.1521/jsyt.2013.32.3.60

Froerer, A. S., von Cziffra-Bergs, J., Kim, J. S., & Connie, E. E. (Eds.). (2018). *Solution-focused brief therapy with clients managing trauma.* Oxford University Press. https://doi.org/10.1093/oso/9780190678784.001.0001

Furman, B. (2010). *Kids skills in action: Stories of playful and practical solution-finding with children.* St. Luke's Innovative Resources.

Furman, B., & Ahola, T. (1992). *Solution talk: Hosting therapeutic conversations.* W. W. Norton.

Gassmann, D., & Grawe, K. (2006). General change mechanisms: The relation between problem activation and resource activation in successful and unsuccessful therapeutic interactions. *Clinical Psychology & Psychotherapy, 13*(1), 1–11. https://doi.org/10.1002/cpp.442

Gergen, K. (2015). *An invitation to social construction* (3rd ed.). Sage. https://doi.org/10.4135/9781473921276

Gillaspy, J. A., & Murphy, J. J. (2012). Incorporating outcome and session rating scales in solution-focused brief therapy. In C. Franklin, T. S. Trepper, W. J. Gingerich, & E. E. McCollum (Eds.), *Solution-focused brief therapy: Research, practice, and training* (pp. 73–93). Oxford University Press.

Gingerich, W. J., & de Shazer, S. (1991). The BRIEFER project: Using expert systems as theory construction tools. *Family Process, 30*(2), 241–250. https://doi.org/10.1111/j.1545-5300.1991.00241.x

Gingerich, W. J., & Eisengart, S. (2000). Solution-focused brief therapy: A review of the outcome research. *Family Process, 39*(4), 477–498. https://doi.org/10.1111/j.1545-5300.2000.39408.x

Gingerich, W. J., Kim, J. S., Stams, G. J. J. M., & Macdonald, A. J. (2012). Solution-focused brief therapy outcome research. In C. Franklin, T. S. Trepper, W. J. Gingerich, & E. E. McCollum (Eds.), *Solution-focused brief therapy: A handbook of evidence-based practice* (pp. 95–111). Oxford University Press.

Gingerich, W. J., & Peterson, L. T. (2013). Effectiveness of solution-focused brief therapy: A systematic qualitative review of controlled outcome studies. *Research on Social Work Practice, 23*(3), 266–283. https://doi.org/10.1177/1049731512470859

Gong, H., & Hsu, W. S. (2017). The effectiveness of solution-focused group therapy in ethnic Chinese school settings: A meta-analysis. *International Journal of Group Psychotherapy, 67*(3), 383–409. https://doi.org/10.1080/00207284.2016.1240588

Gong, H., & Xu, W. (2015). A meta-analysis on the effectiveness of solution-focused brief therapy. *Studies of Psychology and Behavior, 13*(6), 799–803.

Grant, A. M. (2012). Making positive change: A randomized study comparing solution-focused vs. problem-focused coaching questions. *Journal of Systemic Therapies, 31*(2), 21–35. https://doi.org/10.1521/jsyt.2012.31.2.21

Haley, J. (Ed.). (1967). *Advanced techniques of hypnosis and therapy: Selected papers of Milton H. Erickson, M.D.* Grune & Stratton.

Haley, J. (1973). *Uncommon therapy: The psychiatric techniques of Milton H. Erickson, M.D.* W. W. Norton.

Haley, J. (1997). *Leaving home: The therapy of disturbed young people.* Routledge.

Hansen, N. B., & Lambert, M. J. (2003). An evaluation of the dose–response relationship in naturalistic treatment settings using survival analysis. *Mental Health Services Research*, 5(1), 1–12. https://doi.org/10.1023/A:1021751307358

Hendrick, S., Isebaert, L., & Dolan, Y. (2012). Solution-focused brief therapy in alcohol treatment. In C. Franklin, T. S. Trepper, W. J. Gingerich, & E. E. McCollum (Eds.), *Solution-focused brief therapy: A handbook of evidence-based practice* (pp. 264–278). Oxford University Press.

Hook, J. N., Davis, D., Owen, J., & DeBlaere, C. (2017). *Cultural humility: Engaging diverse identities in therapy*. American Psychological Association.

Hook, J. N., Davis, D. E., Owen, J., Worthington, E. L., Jr., & Utsey, S. O. (2013). Cultural humility: Measuring openness to culturally diverse clients. *Journal of Counseling Psychology*, 60(3), 353–366. https://doi.org/10.1037/a0032595

Horvath, A. O., Del Re, A. C., Flückiger, C., & Symonds, D. (2011). Alliance in individual psychotherapy. In J. C. Norcross (Ed.), *Psychotherapy relationships that work: Evidence-based responsiveness* (2nd ed., pp. 25–69). Oxford University Press. https://doi.org/10.1093/acprof:oso/9780199737208.003.0002

Hoyt, M. F., Bobele, M., Slive, A., Young, J., & Talmon, M. (Eds.). (2018). *Single-session therapy by walk-in or appointment: Administrative, clinical, and supervisory aspects of one-at-a-time services*. Routledge. https://doi.org/10.4324/9781351112437

Hubble, M. A., Duncan, B. L., Miller, S. D., & Wampold, B. E. (2010). Introduction. In B. L. Duncan, S. D. Miller, B. E. Wampold, & M. A. Hubble (Eds.), *The heart and soul of change: Delivering what works in therapy* (2nd ed., pp. 23–46). American Psychological Association. https://doi.org/10.1037/12075-001

Iveson, C., George, E., & Ratner, H. (2012). *Brief coaching: A solution focused approach*. Routledge. https://doi.org/10.4324/9780203144411

Ivey, A. E., Ivey, M. B., & Zalaquett, C. P. (2018). *Intentional interviewing and counseling: Facilitating client development in a multicultural society*. Cengage.

Kegel, A. F., & Flückiger, C. (2015). Predicting psychotherapy dropouts: A multilevel approach. *Clinical Psychology & Psychotherapy*, 22(5), 377–386. https://doi.org/10.1002/cpp.1899

Kim, J. S. (2008). Examining the effectiveness of solution-focused brief therapy: A meta-analysis. *Research on Social Work Practice*, 18(2), 107–116. https://doi.org/10.1177/1049731507307807

Kim, J. S. (Ed.). (2014). *Solution-focused brief therapy: A multicultural approach*. Sage. https://doi.org/10.4135/9781483352930

Kim, J. S., Franklin, C., Zhang, Y., Liu, X., Qu, Y., & Chen, H. (2015). Solution-focused brief therapy in China: A meta-analysis. *Journal of Ethnic & Cultural Diversity in Social Work*, 24(3), 187–201. https://doi.org/10.1080/15313204.2014.991983

Kim, J. S., Kelly, M. S., & Franklin, C. (2017). *Solution-focused brief therapy in schools: A 360-degree view of the research and practice principles* (2nd ed.). Oxford University Press. https://doi.org/10.1093/acprof:oso/9780190607258.001.0001

Kim, J. S., Smock, S., Trepper, T. S., McCollum, E. E., & Franklin, C. (2010). Is solution-focused brief therapy evidence-based? *Families in Society, 91*(3), 300–306. https://doi.org/10.1606/1044-3894.4009

Kim, J. S., Smock Jordan, S., Franklin, C., & Froerer, A. (2019). Is solution-focused brief therapy evidence-based? An update 10 years later. *Families in Society, 100*(2), 127–138. https://doi.org/10.1177/1044389419841688

Korman, H. (2004). *The common project.* SIKT. https://solutions-centre.org/pdf/Common_Project1.pdf

Korman, H., Bavelas, J. B., & De Jong, P. (2013). Microanalysis of formulations in solution-focused brief therapy, cognitive behavioral therapy, and motivational interviewing. *Journal of Systemic Therapies, 32*(3), 31–45. https://doi.org/10.1521/jsyt.2013.32.3.31

Korman, H., De Jong, P., & Smock Jordan, S. (2020). Steve de Shazer's theory development. *Journal of Solution Focused Practices, 4*(2), 47–70. https://digitalscholarship.unlv.edu/journalsfp/vol4/iss2/5

Kort, B., Froerer, A., & Walker, C. (2021). Creating a common language: How solution-focused brief therapy reflects current principles of change and common factors. *Journal of Solution-Focused Practices, 5*(1), 30–44. https://digitalscholarship.unlv.edu/journalsfp/vol5/iss1/5

Lambert, M. J. (2013). The efficacy and effectiveness of psychotherapy. In M. J. Lambert (Ed.), *Bergin and Garfield's handbook of psychotherapy and behavior change* (6th ed., pp. 169–218). Wiley.

Lambert, M. J., Whipple, J. L., & Kleinstäuber, M. (2019). Collecting and delivering client feedback. In J. C. Norcross & M. J. Lambert (Eds.), *Psychotherapy relationships that work: Evidence-based therapist contributions* (pp. 580–630). Oxford University Press. https://doi.org/10.1093/med-psych/9780190843953.003.0017

Lankton, S., & Lankton, C. (1983). *The answer within: A clinical framework of Ericksonian hypnotherapy.* Crown House.

Levenson, H. (2017). *Brief dynamic therapy* (2nd ed.). American Psychological Association. https://doi.org/10.1037/0000043-000

Lipchik, E. (2002). *Beyond technique in solution-focused therapy: Working with emotions and the therapeutic relationship.* Guilford Press.

Lipchik, E. (2014). The development of my personal solution-focused working model: From 1978 and continuing. *International Journal of Solution-Focused Practices, 2*(2), 63–73. https://solutions-centre.org/pdf/25-64-1-PB.pdf

Lipchik, E., Derks, J., Lacourt, M., & Nunnally, E. (2012). The evolution of solution-focused brief therapy. In C. Franklin, T. S. Trepper, W. J. Gingerich, & E. E. McCollum (Eds.), *Solution-focused brief therapy: A handbook of evidence-based practice* (pp. 3–19). Oxford University Press.

Macdonald, A. (2011). *Solution-focused therapy: Theory, research and practice* (2nd ed.). Sage. https://doi.org/10.4135/9781446288764

Macdonald, A. (2017). *Solution-focused approaches.* https://solutionsdoc.co.uk/sfbt-evaluation-list/

Madigan, S. (2019). *Narrative therapy* (2nd ed.). American Psychological Association.

McKergow, M. (2021). *The next generation of solution focused practice: Stretching the world for new opportunities and progress.* Routledge. https://doi.org/10.4324/9780367855710

McNamee, S., & Gergen, K. (Eds.). (1992). *Therapy as social construction.* SAGE Publications.

Merriam-Webster. (n.d.). Amplify. In *Merriam-Webster.com dictionary.* Retrieved April 4, 2023, from https://www.merriam-webster.com/dictionary/amplify?utm_campaign=sd&utm_medium=serp&utm_source=jsonld

Miller, S. D., & Duncan, B. L. (2000). *Outcome Rating Scale.* https://blog.betteroutcomesnow.com/ors-and-srs-rating-scales-development

Miller, S. D., Duncan, B. L., & Johnson, L. D. (2002). *Session Rating Scale.* https://blog.betteroutcomesnow.com/ors-and-srs-rating-scales-development

Muran, J. C., Safran, J. D., Gorman, B. S., Samstag, L. W., Eubanks-Carter, C., & Winston, A. (2009). The relationship of early alliance ruptures and their resolution to process and outcome in three time-limited psychotherapies for personality disorders. *Psychotherapy: Theory, Research, Practice, Training, 46*(2), 233–248. https://doi.org/10.1037/a0016085

Murphy, J. J. (2023). *Solution-focused counseling in schools* (4th ed.). American Counseling Association.

Murphy, J. J., & Duncan, B. L. (2007). *Brief intervention for school problems: Outcome-informed strategies* (2nd ed.). Guilford Press.

Murphy, J. J., & Sparks, J. A. (2018). *Strengths-based therapy.* Routledge. https://doi.org/10.4324/9781315512976

Neipp, M. C., & Beyebach, M. (2022). The global outcomes of solution-focused brief therapy: A revision. *The American Journal of Family Therapy.* https://doi.org/10.1080/01926187.2022.2069175

Neipp, M. C., Beyebach, M., Nuñez, R. M., & Martínez-González, M. C. (2016). The effect of solution-focused versus problem-focused questions: A replication. *Journal of Marital and Family Therapy, 42*(3), 525–535. https://doi.org/10.1111/jmft.12140

Ness, M. E., & Murphy, J. J. (2001). Pretreatment change by clients in a university counseling center: Relationship to inquiry technique, client, and situational variables. *Journal of College Counseling, 4*(1), 20–31. https://doi.org/10.1002/j.2161-1882.2001.tb00180.x

Nissen-Lie, H. A., Rønnestad, M. H., Høglend, P. A., Havik, O. E., Solbakken, O. A., Stiles, T. C., & Monsen, J. T. (2017). Love yourself as a person, doubt yourself as a therapist? *Clinical Psychology & Psychotherapy, 24*(1), 48–60. https://doi.org/10.1002/cpp.1977

Norcross, J. C., & Lambert, M. J. (2019). Evidence-based psychotherapy relationship: The third task force. In J. C. Norcross & M. J. Lambert (Eds.), *Psychotherapy relationships that work: Evidence-based therapist contributions* (3rd ed., pp. 1–23). Oxford University Press.

Norcross, J. C., & Wampold, B. E. (2019). Relationships and responsiveness in the psychological treatment of trauma: The tragedy of the APA Clinical Practice Guideline. *Psychotherapy, 56*(3), 391–399. https://doi.org/10.1037/pst0000228

Nylund, D., & Corsiglia, V. (1994). Being solution-focused forced in brief therapy: Remembering something important we already knew. *Journal of Systemic Therapies, 13*(1), 5–12. https://doi.org/10.1521/jsyt.1994.13.1.5

O'Hanlon, B., & Bertolino, B. (2002). *Even from a broken web: Brief, respectful solution-oriented therapy for sexual abuse and trauma.* Wiley.

O'Hanlon, B., & Weiner-Davis, M. (2003). *In search of solutions: A new direction in psychotherapy* (Rev. ed.). W. W. Norton.

Oregon Health Authority. (2017). *Addictions and Mental Health Services.* https://www.oregon.gov/oha/hsd/amh/pages/ebp-practices.aspx?wp3699=p:7#g_

Panayotov, P. A., Strahilov, B. E., & Anichkina, A. Y. (2012). Solution-focused brief therapy and medication adherence with schizophrenic patients. In C. Franklin, T. S. Trepper, W. J. Gingerich, & E. E. McCollum (Eds.), *Solution-focused brief therapy: A handbook of evidence-based practice* (pp. 196–202). Oxford University Press.

Pichot, T., & Dolan, Y. M. (2003). *Solution-focused brief therapy: Its effective use in agency settings.* Routledge.

Pichot, T., & Smock, S. A. (2009). *Solution-focused substance abuse treatment.* Routledge.

Price, M., Polk, W., Hill, N. E., Liang, B., & Perella, J. (2019). The intersectionality of identity-based victimization in adolescence: A person-centered examination of mental health and academic achievement in a U.S. high school. *Journal of Adolescence, 76*(1), 185–196. https://doi.org/10.1016/j.adolescence.2019.09.002

Prochaska, J. O., Norcross, J. C., & DiClemente, C. C. (1994). *Changing for good.* William Morrow.

Ratner, H., George, E., & Iveson, C. (2012). *Solution-focused brief therapy: 100 key points and techniques.* Routledge. https://doi.org/10.4324/9780203116562

Ratner, H., & Yusuf, D. (2015). *Brief coaching with children and young people.* Routledge. https://doi.org/10.4324/9781315743684

Ridley, C. R. (2005). *Overcoming unintentional racism in counseling and therapy: A practitioner's guide to intentional intervention* (2nd ed.). SAGE. https://doi.org/10.4135/9781452204468

Rogers, C. R. (1957). The necessary and sufficient conditions of therapeutic personality change. *Journal of Consulting Psychology, 21*(2), 95–103. https://doi.org/10.1037/h0045357

Rosenzweig, S. (1936). Some implicit common factors in diverse methods of psychotherapy. *American Journal of Orthopsychiatry, 6*(3), 412–415. https://doi.org/10.1111/j.1939-0025.1936.tb05248.x

Schlanger, K., Pascual-Sánchez, A., Díaz Arnal, G., & Torralba Viorreta, R. (2019). MRI/problem-solving brief therapy: The evolution of the model as illustrated in the case of an adolescent girl that proves difficult for the therapist. *Journal of Systemic Therapies, 38*(2), 47–63. https://doi.org/10.1521/jsyt.2019.38.2.47

Selekman, M. D. (2009). *The adolescent and young adult self-harming treatment manual.* W. W. Norton.

Seligman, M. E. P. (1998). Building human strengths: Psychology's forgotten mission. *APA Monitor, 28*(1), 2. (See the shaded box in this link for APA Monitor article: https://www.sagepub.com/sites/default/files/upm-binaries/11232_Chapter_1.pdf)

Shapiro, J. P., Friedberg, R. D., & Bardenstein, K. K. (2006). *Child and adolescent therapy: Science and art.* Wiley.

Shennan, G. (2019). *Solution-focused practice: Effective communication to facilitate change* (2nd ed.). Red Globe Press.

Short, D., Erickson, B. A., & Erickson Klein, R. (2005). *Hope and resiliency: Understanding the psychotherapeutic strategies of Milton H. Erickson, M.D.* Crown House.

Simon, J. K., & Nelson, T. S. (2007). *Solution-focused brief practice with long-term clients in mental health services: I am more than my label.* Routledge.

Smith, I. C. (Ed.). (2006). Riding the underground railroad: Insoo Kim Berg talks about the origins and future of the solution-focused approach. *Solution News, 2*(3), 3–6. https://paperzz.com/doc/8572672/riding-the-underground-railroad%E2%80%A6

Smock, S. A., McCollum, E. E., & Stevenson, M. L. (2010). The development of the solution building inventory. *Journal of Marital and Family Therapy, 36*(4), 499–510. https://doi.org/10.1111/j.1752-0606.2010.00197.x

Smock Jordan, S., Froerer, A. S., & Bavelas, J. B. (2013). Microanalysis of positive and negative content in solution-focused brief therapy and cognitive behavioral therapy expert sessions. *Journal of Systemic Therapies, 32*(3), 46–59. https://doi.org/10.1521/jsyt.2013.32.3.46

Sobhy, M., & Cavallaro, M. (2010). Solution-focused brief counseling in schools: Theoretical perspectives and case application to an elementary school student. *VISTAS Online,* Article 81. https://www.counseling.org/resources/library/vistas/2010-v-online/article_81.pdf

Sommers-Flanagan, J., & Sommers-Flanagan, R. (2018). *Counseling and psychotherapy theories in context and practice: Skills, strategies, and techniques* (3rd ed.). Wiley.

Sue, D. W., Sue, D., Neville, H. A., & Smith, L. (2019). *Counseling the culturally diverse: Theory and practice* (8th ed.). Wiley.

Sue, S., & Zane, N. (2006). Ethnic minority populations have been neglected by evidence-based practices. In J. C. Norcross, L. E. Beutler, & R. F. Levant (Eds.), *Evidence-based practices in mental health: Debate and dialogue on the fundamental questions* (pp. 338–345). American Psychological Association.

Terlizzi, E. P., & Schiller, J. S. (2022). *Mental health treatment among adults aged 18–44: United States, 2019–2021* (NCHS Data Brief 444). National Center for Health Statistics. https://www.cdc.gov/nchs/products/databriefs/db444.htm

Thomas, F. N. (2013). *Solution-focused supervision: A resource-oriented approach to developing clinical expertise.* Springer. https://doi.org/10.1007/978-1-4614-6052-7

Trepper, T. S., & Franklin, C. (2012). Epilogue. In C. Franklin, T. S. Trepper, W. J. Gingerich, & E. E. McCollum (Eds.), *Solution-focused brief therapy: A handbook of evidence-based practice* (pp. 405–412). Oxford University Press.

Tryon, G. S., Birch, S. E., & Verkuilen, J. (2019). Goal consensus and collaboration. In J. C. Norcross & M. J. Lambert (Eds.), *Psychotherapy relationships that work: Vol. 1. Evidence-based therapist contributions* (3rd ed., pp. 167–204). Oxford University Press. https://doi.org/10.1093/med-psych/9780190843953.003.0005

Vaihinger, H. (1924). *The philosophy of "as if": A system of the theoretical, practical and religious fictions of mankind* (C. K. Ogden, Trans.). Routledge.

VandenBos, G. R. (Ed.). (2015). *APA dictionary of psychology* (2nd ed.). American Psychological Association. https://doi.org/10.1037/14646-000

von Bertalanffy, L. (1968). *General systems theory: Foundations, development, applications.* George Braziller.

Wampold, B. E., & Imel, Z. E. (2015). *The great psychotherapy debate: The evidence for what makes psychotherapy work* (2nd ed.). Routledge. https://doi.org/10.4324/9780203582015

Watzlawick, P., Bavelas, J. B., & Jackson, D. D. (1967). *Pragmatics of human communication: A study of interactional patterns, pathologies and paradoxes.* W. W. Norton.

Watzlawick, P., Weakland, J. H., & Fisch, R. (1974). *Change: Principles of problem formation and problem resolution.* W. W. Norton.

Weakland, J. H. (1993). Conversation—But what kind? In S. G. Gilligan & R. Price (Eds.), *Therapeutic conversations* (pp. 136–145). W. W. Norton.

Weiner, N. (1948). *Cybernetics: Or control and communication in the animal and the machine.* Wiley.

Weiner-Davis, M. (1992). *Divorce busting: A step-by-step approach to making your marriage loving again.* Simon & Shuster.

Weiner-Davis, M., de Shazer, S., & Gingerich, W. (1987). Building on pretreatment change to construct a therapeutic solution: An exploratory study. *Journal of Marital and Family Therapy, 13*(4), 359–363. https://doi.org/10.1111/j.1752-0606.1987.tb00717.x

White, M., & Epston, D. (1990). *Narrative means to therapeutic ends.* W. W. Norton.

Wierzbicki, M., & Pekarik, G. (1993). A meta-analysis of psychotherapy dropout. *Professional Psychology, Research and Practice, 24*(2), 190–195. https://doi.org/10.1037/0735-7028.24.2.190

Wittgenstein, L. (1953). *Philosophical investigations.* Macmillan.

Zak, A. M. (2022). What is helpful: The client's perception of the solution-focused brief therapy process by level of engagement. *Journal of Solution Focused Practices, 6*(2), 4–22. https://digitalscholarship.unlv.edu/journalsfp/vol6/iss2/5

Zeig, J. K. (Ed.). (1982). *Ericksonian approaches to hypnosis and psychotherapy.* Bruner/Mazel.

Zhai, Y., & Zhu, Y. (2016). Study of effect on solution-focused approach in improving the negative emotion of surgical patients in department of vascular surgery. *Pakistan Journal of Pharmaceutical Sciences, 29*(2, Suppl.), 719–722. PMID: 27113302. https://applications.emro.who.int/imemrf/Pak_J_Pharm_Sci/Pak_J_Pharm_Sci_2016_29_2suppl_719_722.pdf

Index

About the Author

John J. Murphy, PhD, is a licensed psychologist and Professor Emeritus at the University of Central Arkansas. He completed his PhD in school psychology from the University of Cincinnati and postdoctoral work in client-directed psychotherapy with Barry Duncan at the Dayton (Ohio) Institute for Family Therapy. Dr. Murphy has worked as a high school teacher, school psychologist, and psychotherapist in private practice, where he continues to offer in-person and teletherapy services to clients of all ages. He was previously named one of the top five school psychologists in the United States by the National Association of School Psychologists, and his book *Solution-Focused Counseling in Schools* (currently in its fourth edition) was voted Best Book of the Year by the American School Counselor Association.

Dr. Murphy has other books on client-directed services for children, adolescents, adults, and families, including *Strengths-Based Therapy* (with Jacqueline A. Sparks) and *Brief Intervention for School Problems* (with Barry L. Duncan). His books have been translated into multiple languages, and his work has been featured in psychotherapy textbooks, *The New York Times* bestseller *Switch, Fast Company* magazine, and the DVD training series *Child Therapy With the Experts.* He has received numerous awards for his clinical work, advocacy efforts, and scholarly publications, including the 2018 Admired Scholar Award from the Society for Personality and Social Psychology. He is a consultant and trainer for the North American Chinese Psychological Association (NACPA) and a project director with the Heart & Soul of Change Project, an international research/advocacy group that promotes respectful, client-directed services for marginalized and underrepresented persons and groups. He is a popular keynote and workshop speaker who has offered classes and workshops throughout the United States and overseas for thousands of mental health practitioners and laypersons. His workshops are known for their practicality and passion for helping people change with dignity. Visit Dr. Murphy's website (https://www.drjohnmurphy.com) to learn more about workshop offerings and other aspects of his work.

About the Series Editor

Matt Englar-Carlson, PhD, is a professor of counseling and director of the Center for Boys and Men at California State University–Fullerton. A Fellow of the American Psychological Association (APA), Dr. Englar-Carlson's scholarship focuses on training helping professionals to work more effectively with boys and men across the full range of human diversity. His publications and presentations are focused on men and masculinities, social justice and diversity issues in psychological training and practice, and theories of psychotherapy. Dr. Englar-Carlson coedited the books *In the Room With Men: A Casebook of Therapeutic Change, Counseling Troubled Boys: A Guidebook for Professionals, Beyond the 50-Minute Hour: Therapists Involved in Meaningful Social Action*, and *A Counselor's Guide to Working With Men*, and he was featured in the APA-produced video *Engaging Men in Psychotherapy*. He was named Researcher of the Year, Professional of the Year, and he received the Professional Service award from the Society for the Psychological Study of Men and Masculinities, and was one of the core authors of the *APA Guidelines for Professional Psychological Practice With Boys and Men*. As a clinician, Dr. Englar-Carlson has worked with children, adults, and families in school, community, and university mental health settings. He is the coauthor of *Adlerian Psychotherapy*, which is part of the Theories of Psychotherapy Series.